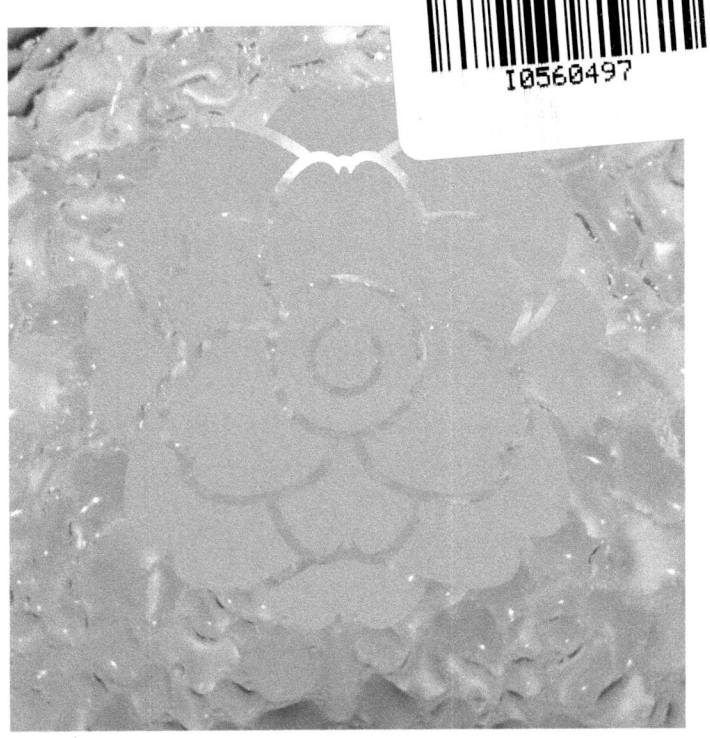

GRATITUDE

JOURNAL

WITH NOTES

GRATITUDE JOURNAL WITH NOTES

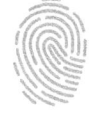

THIS IS THE SOUL PROPERTY

OF _____

Day 1:

Date: _____

Mood: _____

Gratitude:

-
-
- _____

Today's Highlights:

-
- _____

Challenges or Struggles:

-
- _____

What I Learned Today:

-
- _____

Dreams:

-
- _____

Goals for Tomorrow:

-
- _____

Quote of the Day:

- _____

Day 2:

Date: _____

Mood: _____

Gratitude:

-
-
-     _____

Today's Highlights:

-
-     _____

Challenges or Struggles:

-
-     _____

What I Learned Today:

-
-     _____

Dreams:

-
-     _____

Goals for Tomorrow:

-
-     _____

Quote of the Day:

-     _____

Day 3:

Date: _____
Mood: _____

Gratitude:

-
-
- _____

Today's Highlights:

-
- _____

Challenges or Struggles:

-
- _____

What I Learned Today:

-
- _____

Dreams:

-
- _____

Goals for Tomorrow:

-
- _____

Quote of the Day:

- _____

Day 4:

Date: _____

Mood: _____

Gratitude:

-
-
-    _____

Today's Highlights:

-
-    _____

Challenges or Struggles:

-
-    _____

What I Learned Today:

-
-    _____

Dreams:

-
-    _____

Goals for Tomorrow:

-
-    _____

Quote of the Day:

-    _____

Day 5:

Date: _____

Mood: _____

Gratitude:

-
-
- _____

Today's Highlights:

-
- _____

Challenges or Struggles:

-
- _____

What I Learned Today:

-
- _____

Dreams:

-
- _____

Goals for Tomorrow:

-
- _____

Quote of the Day:

- _____

Day 6:

Date: _____

Mood: _____

Gratitude:

-
-
- _____

Today's Highlights:

-
- _____

Challenges or Struggles:

-
- _____

What I Learned Today:

-
- _____

Dreams:

-
- _____

Goals for Tomorrow:

-
- _____

Quote of the Day:

- _____

Day 7:

Date: _____

Mood: _____

Gratitude:

-
-
- _____

Today's Highlights:

-
- _____

Challenges or Struggles:

-
- _____

What I Learned Today:

-
- _____

Dreams:

-
- _____

Goals for Tomorrow:

-
- _____

Quote of the Day:

- _____

Day 8:

Date: _____

Mood: _____

Gratitude:

-
-
- _____

Today's Highlights:

-
- _____

Challenges or Struggles:

-
- _____

What I Learned Today:

-
- _____

Dreams:

-
- _____

Goals for Tomorrow:

-
- _____

Quote of the Day:

- _____

Day 9:

Date: _____

Mood: _____

Gratitude:

-
-
- _____

Today's Highlights:

-
- _____

Challenges or Struggles:

-
- _____

What I Learned Today:

-
- _____

Dreams:

-
- _____

Goals for Tomorrow:

-
- _____

Quote of the Day:

- _____

Day 10:

Date: _____

Mood: _____

Gratitude:

-
-
-     _____

Today's Highlights:

-
-     _____

Challenges or Struggles:

-
-     _____

What I Learned Today:

-
-     _____

Dreams:

-
-     _____

Goals for Tomorrow:

-
-     _____

Quote of the Day:

-     _____

Day 11:

Date: _____

Mood: _____

Gratitude:

-
-
-    _____

Today's Highlights:

-
-    _____

Challenges or Struggles:

-
-    _____

What I Learned Today:

-
-    _____

Dreams:

-
-    _____

Goals for Tomorrow:

-
-    _____

Quote of the Day:

-    _____

Day 12:

Date: _____

Mood: _____

Gratitude:

-
-
- _____

Today's Highlights:

-
- _____

Challenges or Struggles:

-
- _____

What I Learned Today:

-
- _____

Dreams:

-
- _____

Goals for Tomorrow:

-
- _____

Quote of the Day:

- _____

Day 13:

Date: _____

Mood: _____

Gratitude:

-
-
- _____

Today's Highlights:

-
- _____

Challenges or Struggles:

-
- _____

What I Learned Today:

-
- _____

Dreams:

-
- _____

Goals for Tomorrow:

-
- _____

Quote of the Day:

- _____

Day 14:

Date: _____

Mood: _____

Gratitude:

-
-
- _____

Today's Highlights:

-
- _____

Challenges or Struggles:

-
- _____

What I Learned Today:

-
- _____

Dreams:

-
- _____

Goals for Tomorrow:

-
- _____

Quote of the Day:

- _____

Day 15:

Date: _____

Mood: _____

Gratitude:

-
-
- _____

Today's Highlights:

-
- _____

Challenges or Struggles:

-
- _____

What I Learned Today:

-
- _____

Dreams:

-
- _____

Goals for Tomorrow:

-
- _____

Quote of the Day:

- _____

Day 16:

Date: _____

Mood: _____

Gratitude:

-
-
-   _____

Today's Highlights:

-
-   _____

Challenges or Struggles:

-
-   _____

What I Learned Today:

-
-   _____

Dreams:

-
-   _____

Goals for Tomorrow:

-
-   _____

Quote of the Day:

-   _____

Day 17:

Date: _____

Mood: _____

Gratitude:

-
-
- _____

Today's Highlights:

-
- _____

Challenges or Struggles:

-
- _____

What I Learned Today:

-
- _____

Dreams:

-
- _____

Goals for Tomorrow:

-
- _____

Quote of the Day:

- _____

Day 18:

Date: _____

Mood: _____

Gratitude:

-
-
-    _____

Today's Highlights:

-
-    _____

Challenges or Struggles:

-
-    _____

What I Learned Today:

-
-    _____

Dreams:

-
-    _____

Goals for Tomorrow:

-
-    _____

Quote of the Day:

-    _____
-

Day 19:

Date: _____

Mood: _____

Gratitude:

-
-
- _____

Today's Highlights:

-
- _____

Challenges or Struggles:

-
- _____

What I Learned Today:

-
- _____

Dreams:

-
- _____

Goals for Tomorrow:

-
- _____

Quote of the Day:

- _____

Day 20:

Date: _____

Mood: _____

Gratitude:

-
-
- _____

Today's Highlights:

-
- _____

Challenges or Struggles:

-
- _____

What I Learned Today:

-
- _____

Dreams:

-
- _____

Goals for Tomorrow:

-
- _____

Quote of the Day:

- _____

Day 21:

Date: _____

Mood: _____

Gratitude:

-
-
- _____

Today's Highlights:

-
- _____

Challenges or Struggles:

-
- _____

What I Learned Today:

-
- _____

Dreams:

-
- _____

Goals for Tomorrow:

-
- _____

Quote of the Day:

- _____

Day 22:

Date: _____
Mood: _____

Gratitude:

-
-
-        _____

Today's Highlights:

-
-        _____

Challenges or Struggles:

-
-        _____

What I Learned Today:

-
-        _____

Dreams:

-
-        _____

Goals for Tomorrow:

-
-        _____

Quote of the Day:

-        _____

Day 23:

Date: _____

Mood: _____

Gratitude:

-
-
- _____

Today's Highlights:

-
- _____

Challenges or Struggles:

-
- _____

What I Learned Today:

-
- _____

Dreams:

-
- _____

Goals for Tomorrow:

-
- _____

Quote of the Day:

- _____

Day 24:

Date: _____

Mood: _____

Gratitude:

-
-
-   _____

Today's Highlights:

-
-   _____

Challenges or Struggles:

-
-   _____

What I Learned Today:

-
-   _____

Dreams:

-
-   _____

Goals for Tomorrow:

-
-   _____

Quote of the Day:

-   _____

Day 25:

Date: _____

Mood: _____

Gratitude:

-
-
- _____

Today's Highlights:

-
- _____

Challenges or Struggles:

-
- _____

What I Learned Today:

-
- _____

Dreams:

-
- _____

Goals for Tomorrow:

-
- _____

Quote of the Day:

- _____

Day 26:

Date: _____

Mood: _____

Gratitude:

-
-
- _____

Today's Highlights:

-
- _____

Challenges or Struggles:

-
- _____

What I Learned Today:

-
- _____

Dreams:

-
- _____

Goals for Tomorrow:

-
- _____

Quote of the Day:

- _____

Day 27:

Date: _____

Mood: _____

Gratitude:

-
-
- _____

Today's Highlights:

-
- _____

Challenges or Struggles:

-
- _____

What I Learned Today:

-
- _____

Dreams:

-
- _____

Goals for Tomorrow:

-
- _____

Quote of the Day:

- _____

Day 28:

Date: _____

Mood: _____

Gratitude:

-
-
- _____

Today's Highlights:

-
- _____

Challenges or Struggles:

-
- _____

What I Learned Today:

-
- _____

Dreams:

-
- _____

Goals for Tomorrow:

-
- _____

Quote of the Day:

- _____

Day 29:

Date: _____

Mood: _____

Gratitude:

-
-
- _____

Today's Highlights:

-
- _____

Challenges or Struggles:

-
- _____

What I Learned Today:

-
- _____

Dreams:

-
- _____

Goals for Tomorrow:

-
- _____

Quote of the Day:

- _____

Day 30:

Date: _____

Mood: _____

Gratitude:

-
-
- _____

Today's Highlights:

-
- _____

Challenges or Struggles:

-
- _____

What I Learned Today:

-
- _____

Dreams:

-
- _____

Goals for Tomorrow:

-
- _____

Quote of the Day:

- _____

Day 31:

Date: _____

Mood: _____

Gratitude:

-
-
- _____

Today's Highlights:

-
- _____

Challenges or Struggles:

-
- _____

What I Learned Today:

-
- _____

Dreams:

-
- _____

Goals for Tomorrow:

-
- _____

Quote of the Day:

- _____

Day 32:

Date: _____

Mood: _____

Gratitude:

-
-
- _____

Today's Highlights:

-
- _____

Challenges or Struggles:

-
- _____

What I Learned Today:

-
- _____

Dreams:

-
- _____

Goals for Tomorrow:

-
- _____

Quote of the Day:

- _____

Day 33:

Date: _____
Mood: _____

Gratitude:

-
-
- _____

Today's Highlights:

-
- _____

Challenges or Struggles:

-
- _____

What I Learned Today:

-
- _____

Dreams:

-
- _____

Goals for Tomorrow:

-
- _____

Quote of the Day:

- _____

Day 34:

Date: _____

Mood: _____

Gratitude:

-
-
- _____

Today's Highlights:

-
- _____

Challenges or Struggles:

-
- _____

What I Learned Today:

-
- _____

Dreams:

-
- _____

Goals for Tomorrow:

-
- _____

Quote of the Day:

- _____

Day 35:

Date: _____

Mood: _____

Gratitude:

-
-
- _____

Today's Highlights:

-
- _____

Challenges or Struggles:

-
- _____

What I Learned Today:

-
- _____

Dreams:

-
- _____

Goals for Tomorrow:

-
- _____

Quote of the Day:

- _____

Day 36:

Date: _____

Mood: _____

Gratitude:

-
-
- _____

Today's Highlights:

-
- _____

Challenges or Struggles:

-
- _____

What I Learned Today:

-
- _____

Dreams:

-
- _____

Goals for Tomorrow:

-
- _____

Quote of the Day:

- _____

Day 37:

Date: _____

Mood: _____

Gratitude:

-
-
- _____

Today's Highlights:

-
- _____

Challenges or Struggles:

-
- _____

What I Learned Today:

-
- _____

Dreams:

-
- _____

Goals for Tomorrow:

-
- _____

Quote of the Day:

- _____

Day 38:

Date: _____

Mood: _____

Gratitude:

-
-
- _____

Today's Highlights:

-
- _____

Challenges or Struggles:

-
- _____

What I Learned Today:

-
- _____

Dreams:

-
- _____

Goals for Tomorrow:

-
- _____

Quote of the Day:

- _____

Day 39:

Date: _____

Mood: _____

Gratitude:

-
-
- _____

Today's Highlights:

-
- _____

Challenges or Struggles:

-
- _____

What I Learned Today:

-
- _____

Dreams:

-
- _____

Goals for Tomorrow:

-
- _____

Quote of the Day:

- _____

Day 40:

Date: _____

Mood: _____

Gratitude:

-
-
- _____

Today's Highlights:

-
- _____

Challenges or Struggles:

-
- _____

What I Learned Today:

-
- _____

Dreams:

-
- _____

Goals for Tomorrow:

-
- _____

Quote of the Day:

- _____

Day 41:

Date: _____

Mood: _____

Gratitude:

-
-
-     _____

Today's Highlights:

-
-     _____

Challenges or Struggles:

-
-     _____

What I Learned Today:

-
-     _____

Dreams:

-
-     _____

Goals for Tomorrow:

-
-     _____

Quote of the Day:

-     _____

Day 42:

Date: _____

Mood: _____

Gratitude:

-
-
- _____

Today's Highlights:

-
- _____

Challenges or Struggles:

-
- _____

What I Learned Today:

-
- _____

Dreams:

-
- _____

Goals for Tomorrow:

-
- _____

Quote of the Day:

- _____

Day 43:

Date: _____

Mood: _____

Gratitude:

-
-
- _____

Today's Highlights:

-
- _____

Challenges or Struggles:

-
- _____

What I Learned Today:

-
- _____

Dreams:

-
- _____

Goals for Tomorrow:

-
- _____

Quote of the Day:

- _____

Day 44:

Date: _____

Mood: _____

Gratitude:

-
-
-    _____

Today's Highlights:

-
-    _____

Challenges or Struggles:

-
-    _____

What I Learned Today:

-
-    _____

Dreams:

-
-    _____

Goals for Tomorrow:

-
-    _____

Quote of the Day:

-    _____

Day 45:

Date: _____

Mood: _____

Gratitude:

-
-
- _____

Today's Highlights:

-
- _____

Challenges or Struggles:

-
- _____

What I Learned Today:

-
- _____

Dreams:

-
- _____

Goals for Tomorrow:

-
- _____

Quote of the Day:

- _____

Day 46:

Date: _____

Mood: _____

Gratitude:

-
-
-    _____

Today's Highlights:

-
-    _____

Challenges or Struggles:

-
-    _____

What I Learned Today:

-
-    _____

Dreams:

-
-    _____

Goals for Tomorrow:

-
-    _____

Quote of the Day:

-    _____

Day 47:

Date: _____

Mood: _____

Gratitude:

-
-
- _____

Today's Highlights:

-
- _____

Challenges or Struggles:

-
- _____

What I Learned Today:

-
- _____

Dreams:

-
- _____

Goals for Tomorrow:

-
- _____

Quote of the Day:

- _____

Day 48:

Date: _____

Mood: _____

Gratitude:

-
-
- _____

Today's Highlights:

-
- _____

Challenges or Struggles:

-
- _____

What I Learned Today:

-
- _____

Dreams:

-
- _____

Goals for Tomorrow:

-
- _____

Quote of the Day:

- _____

Day 49:

Date: _____

Mood: _____

Gratitude:

-
-
-     _____

Today's Highlights:

-
-     _____

Challenges or Struggles:

-
-     _____

What I Learned Today:

-
-     _____

Dreams:

-
-     _____

Goals for Tomorrow:

-
-     _____

Quote of the Day:

-     _____

Day 50:

Date: _____

Mood: _____

Gratitude:

-
-
- _____

Today's Highlights:

-
- _____

Challenges or Struggles:

-
- _____

What I Learned Today:

-
- _____

Dreams:

-
- _____

Goals for Tomorrow:

-
- _____

Quote of the Day:

- _____

Day 51:

Date: _____

Mood: _____

Gratitude:

-
-
- _____

Today's Highlights:

-
- _____

Challenges or Struggles:

-
- _____

What I Learned Today:

-
- _____

Dreams:

-
- _____

Goals for Tomorrow:

-
- _____

Quote of the Day:

- _____

Day 52:

Date: _____

Mood: _____

Gratitude:

-
-
-    _____

Today's Highlights:

-
-    _____

Challenges or Struggles:

-
-    _____

What I Learned Today:

-
-    _____

Dreams:

-
-    _____

Goals for Tomorrow:

-
-    _____

Quote of the Day:

-    _____

Day 53:

Date: _____

Mood: _____

Gratitude:

-
-
- _____

Today's Highlights:

-
- _____

Challenges or Struggles:

-
- _____

What I Learned Today:

-
- _____

Dreams:

-
- _____

Goals for Tomorrow:

-
- _____

Quote of the Day:

- _____

Day 54:

Date: _____

Mood: _____

Gratitude:

-
-
- _____

Today's Highlights:

-
- _____

Challenges or Struggles:

-
- _____

What I Learned Today:

-
- _____

Dreams:

-
- _____

Goals for Tomorrow:

-
- _____

Quote of the Day:

- _____
-

Day 55:

Date: _____

Mood: _____

Gratitude:

-
-
- _____

Today's Highlights:

-
- _____

Challenges or Struggles:

-
- _____

What I Learned Today:

-
- _____

Dreams:

-
- _____

Goals for Tomorrow:

-
- _____

Quote of the Day:

- _____

Day 56:

Date: _____

Mood: _____

Gratitude:

-
-
- _____

Today's Highlights:

-
- _____

Challenges or Struggles:

-
- _____

What I Learned Today:

-
- _____

Dreams:

-
- _____

Goals for Tomorrow:

-
- _____

Quote of the Day:

- _____

Day 57:

Date: _____

Mood: _____

Gratitude:

-
-
- _____

Today's Highlights:

-
- _____

Challenges or Struggles:

-
- _____

What I Learned Today:

-
- _____

Dreams:

-
- _____

Goals for Tomorrow:

-
- _____

Quote of the Day:

- _____

Day 58:

Date: _____

Mood: _____

Gratitude:

-
-
- _____

Today's Highlights:

-
- _____

Challenges or Struggles:

-
- _____

What I Learned Today:

-
- _____

Dreams:

-
- _____

Goals for Tomorrow:

-
- _____

Quote of the Day:

- _____

Day 59:

Date: _____

Mood: _____

Gratitude:

-
-
- _____

Today's Highlights:

-
- _____

Challenges or Struggles:

-
- _____

What I Learned Today:

-
- _____

Dreams:

-
- _____

Goals for Tomorrow:

-
- _____

Quote of the Day:

- _____

Day 60:

Date: _____

Mood: _____

Gratitude:

-
-
- _____

Today's Highlights:

-
- _____

Challenges or Struggles:

-
- _____

What I Learned Today:

-
- _____

Dreams:

-
- _____

Goals for Tomorrow:

-
- _____

Quote of the Day:

- _____

Day 61:

Date: _____

Mood: _____

Gratitude:

-
-
- _____

Today's Highlights:

-
- _____

Challenges or Struggles:

-
- _____

What I Learned Today:

-
- _____

Dreams:

-
- _____

Goals for Tomorrow:

-
- _____

Quote of the Day:

- _____

Day 62:

Date: _____

Mood: _____

Gratitude:

-
-
-     _____

Today's Highlights:

-
-     _____

Challenges or Struggles:

-
-     _____

What I Learned Today:

-
-     _____

Dreams:

-
-     _____

Goals for Tomorrow:

-
-     _____

Quote of the Day:

-     _____

Day 63:

Date: _____

Mood: _____

Gratitude:

-
-
- _____

Today's Highlights:

-
- _____

Challenges or Struggles:

-
- _____

What I Learned Today:

-
- _____

Dreams:

-
- _____

Goals for Tomorrow:

-
- _____

Quote of the Day:

- _____

Day 64:

Date: _____

Mood: _____

Gratitude:

-
-
-   _____

Today's Highlights:

-
-   _____

Challenges or Struggles:

-
-   _____

What I Learned Today:

-
-   _____

Dreams:

-
-   _____

Goals for Tomorrow:

-
-   _____

Quote of the Day:

-   _____

Day 65:

Date: _____

Mood: _____

Gratitude:

-
-
-     _____

Today's Highlights:

-
-     _____

Challenges or Struggles:

-
-     _____

What I Learned Today:

-
-     _____

Dreams:

-
-     _____

Goals for Tomorrow:

-
-     _____

Quote of the Day:

-     _____

Day 66:

Date: _____

Mood: _____

Gratitude:

-
-
-     _____

Today's Highlights:

-
-     _____

Challenges or Struggles:

-
-     _____

What I Learned Today:

-
-     _____

Dreams:

-
-     _____

Goals for Tomorrow:

-
-     _____

Quote of the Day:

-     _____

Day 67:

Date: _____

Mood: _____

Gratitude:

-
-
- _____

Today's Highlights:

-
- _____

Challenges or Struggles:

-
- _____

What I Learned Today:

-
- _____

Dreams:

-
- _____

Goals for Tomorrow:

-
- _____

Quote of the Day:

- _____

Day 68:

Date: _____

Mood: _____

Gratitude:

-
-
- _____

Today's Highlights:

-
- _____

Challenges or Struggles:

-
- _____

What I Learned Today:

-
- _____

Dreams:

-
- _____

Goals for Tomorrow:

-
- _____

Quote of the Day:

- _____

Day 69:

Date: _____

Mood: _____

Gratitude:

-
-
- _____

Today's Highlights:

-
- _____

Challenges or Struggles:

-
- _____

What I Learned Today:

-
- _____

Dreams:

-
- _____

Goals for Tomorrow:

-
- _____

Quote of the Day:

- _____

Day 70:

Date: _____

Mood: _____

Gratitude:

-
-
- _____

Today's Highlights:

-
- _____

Challenges or Struggles:

-
- _____

What I Learned Today:

-
- _____

Dreams:

-
- _____

Goals for Tomorrow:

-
- _____

Quote of the Day:

- _____

Day 71:

Date: _____

Mood: _____

Gratitude:

-
-
- _____

Today's Highlights:

-
- _____

Challenges or Struggles:

-
- _____

What I Learned Today:

-
- _____

Dreams:

-
- _____

Goals for Tomorrow:

-
- _____

Quote of the Day:

- _____

Day 72:

Date: _____

Mood: _____

Gratitude:

-
-
- _____

Today's Highlights:

-
- _____

Challenges or Struggles:

-
- _____

What I Learned Today:

-
- _____

Dreams:

-
- _____

Goals for Tomorrow:

-
- _____

Quote of the Day:

- _____

Day 73:

Date: _____

Mood: _____

Gratitude:

-
-
- _____

Today's Highlights:

-
- _____

Challenges or Struggles:

-
- _____

What I Learned Today:

-
- _____

Dreams:

-
- _____

Goals for Tomorrow:

-
- _____

Quote of the Day:

- _____

Day 74:

Date: _____

Mood: _____

Gratitude:

-
-
- _____

Today's Highlights:

-
- _____

Challenges or Struggles:

-
- _____

What I Learned Today:

-
- _____

Dreams:

-
- _____

Goals for Tomorrow:

-
- _____

Quote of the Day:

- _____

Day 75:

Date: _____

Mood: _____

Gratitude:

-
-
- _____

Today's Highlights:

-
- _____

Challenges or Struggles:

-
- _____

What I Learned Today:

-
- _____

Dreams:

-
- _____

Goals for Tomorrow:

-
- _____

Quote of the Day:

- _____

Day 76:

Date: _____

Mood: _____

Gratitude:

-
-
- _____

Today's Highlights:

-
- _____

Challenges or Struggles:

-
- _____

What I Learned Today:

-
- _____

Dreams:

-
- _____

Goals for Tomorrow:

-
- _____

Quote of the Day:

- _____

Day 77:

Date: _____

Mood: _____

Gratitude:

-
-
- _____

Today's Highlights:

-
- _____

Challenges or Struggles:

-
- _____

What I Learned Today:

-
- _____

Dreams:

-
- _____

Goals for Tomorrow:

-
- _____

Quote of the Day:

- _____

Day 78:

Date: _____

Mood: _____

Gratitude:

-
-
- _____

Today's Highlights:

-
- _____

Challenges or Struggles:

-
- _____

What I Learned Today:

-
- _____

Dreams:

-
- _____

Goals for Tomorrow:

-
- _____

Quote of the Day:

- _____

Day 79:

Date: _____

Mood: _____

Gratitude:

-
-
- _____

Today's Highlights:

-
- _____

Challenges or Struggles:

-
- _____

What I Learned Today:

-
- _____

Dreams:

-
- _____

Goals for Tomorrow:

-
- _____

Quote of the Day:

- _____

Day 80:

Date: _____

Mood: _____

Gratitude:

-
-
- _____

Today's Highlights:

-
- _____

Challenges or Struggles:

-
- _____

What I Learned Today:

-
- _____

Dreams:

-
- _____

Goals for Tomorrow:

-
- _____

Quote of the Day:

- _____

Day 81:

Date: _____

Mood: _____

Gratitude:

-
-
- _____

Today's Highlights:

-
- _____

Challenges or Struggles:

-
- _____

What I Learned Today:

-
- _____

Dreams:

-
- _____

Goals for Tomorrow:

-
- _____

Quote of the Day:

- _____

Day 82:

Date: _____

Mood: _____

Gratitude:

-
-
-    _____

Today's Highlights:

-
-    _____

Challenges or Struggles:

-
-    _____

What I Learned Today:

-
-    _____

Dreams:

-
-    _____

Goals for Tomorrow:

-
-    _____

Quote of the Day:

-    _____

Day 83:

Date: _____

Mood: _____

Gratitude:

-
-
- _____

Today's Highlights:

-
- _____

Challenges or Struggles:

-
- _____

What I Learned Today:

-
- _____

Dreams:

-
- _____

Goals for Tomorrow:

-
- _____

Quote of the Day:

- _____

Day 84:

Date: _____

Mood: _____

Gratitude:

-
-
-    _____

Today's Highlights:

-
-    _____

Challenges or Struggles:

-
-    _____

What I Learned Today:

-
-    _____

Dreams:

-
-    _____

Goals for Tomorrow:

-
-    _____

Quote of the Day:

-    _____

Day 85:

Date: _____

Mood: _____

Gratitude:

-
-
- _____

Today's Highlights:

-
- _____

Challenges or Struggles:

-
- _____

What I Learned Today:

-
- _____

Dreams:

-
- _____

Goals for Tomorrow:

-
- _____

Quote of the Day:

- _____

Day 86:

Date: _____

Mood: _____

Gratitude:

-
-
- _____

Today's Highlights:

-
- _____

Challenges or Struggles:

-
- _____

What I Learned Today:

-
- _____

Dreams:

-
- _____

Goals for Tomorrow:

-
- _____

Quote of the Day:

- _____

Day 87:

Date: _____

Mood: _____

Gratitude:

-
-
- _____

Today's Highlights:

-
- _____

Challenges or Struggles:

-
- _____

What I Learned Today:

-
- _____

Dreams:

-
- _____

Goals for Tomorrow:

-
- _____

Quote of the Day:

- _____

Day 88:

Date: _____

Mood: _____

Gratitude:

-
-
-         _____

Today's Highlights:

-
-         _____

Challenges or Struggles:

-
-         _____

What I Learned Today:

-
-         _____

Dreams:

-
-         _____

Goals for Tomorrow:

-
-         _____

Quote of the Day:

-         _____

Day 89:

Date: _____

Mood: _____

Gratitude:

-
-
- _____

Today's Highlights:

-
- _____

Challenges or Struggles:

-
- _____

What I Learned Today:

-
- _____

Dreams:

-
- _____

Goals for Tomorrow:

-
- _____

Quote of the Day:

- _____

Day 90:

Date: _____

Mood: _____

Gratitude:

-
-
-     _____

Today's Highlights:

-
-     _____

Challenges or Struggles:

-
-     _____

What I Learned Today:

-
-     _____

Dreams:

-
-     _____

Goals for Tomorrow:

-
-     _____

Quote of the Day:

-     _____
-

Day 91:

Date: _____

Mood: _____

Gratitude:

-
-
-   _____

Today's Highlights:

-
-   _____

Challenges or Struggles:

-
-   _____

What I Learned Today:

-
-   _____

Dreams:

-
-   _____

Goals for Tomorrow:

-
-   _____

Quote of the Day:

-   _____

Day 92:

Date: _____

Mood: _____

Gratitude:

-
-
- _____

Today's Highlights:

-
- _____

Challenges or Struggles:

-
- _____

What I Learned Today:

-
- _____

Dreams:

-
- _____

Goals for Tomorrow:

-
- _____

Quote of the Day:

- _____

Day 93:

Date: _____

Mood: _____

Gratitude:

-
-
- _____

Today's Highlights:

-
- _____

Challenges or Struggles:

-
- _____

What I Learned Today:

-
- _____

Dreams:

-
- _____

Goals for Tomorrow:

-
- _____

Quote of the Day:

- _____

Day 94:

Date: _____

Mood: _____

Gratitude:

-
-
- _____

Today's Highlights:

-
- _____

Challenges or Struggles:

-
- _____

What I Learned Today:

-
- _____

Dreams:

-
- _____

Goals for Tomorrow:

-
- _____

Quote of the Day:

- _____

Day 95:

Date: _____

Mood: _____

Gratitude:

-
-
- _____

Today's Highlights:

-
- _____

Challenges or Struggles:

-
- _____

What I Learned Today:

-
- _____

Dreams:

-
- _____

Goals for Tomorrow:

-
- _____

Quote of the Day:

- _____

Day 96:

Date: _____

Mood: _____

Gratitude:

-
-
-    _____

Today's Highlights:

-
-    _____

Challenges or Struggles:

-
-    _____

What I Learned Today:

-
-    _____

Dreams:

-
-    _____

Goals for Tomorrow:

-
-    _____

Quote of the Day:

-    _____

Day 97:

Date: _____

Mood: _____

Gratitude:

-
-
- _____

Today's Highlights:

-
- _____

Challenges or Struggles:

-
- _____

What I Learned Today:

-
- _____

Dreams:

-
- _____

Goals for Tomorrow:

-
- _____

Quote of the Day:

- _____

Day 98:

Date: _____

Mood: _____

Gratitude:

-
-
- _____

Today's Highlights:

-
- _____

Challenges or Struggles:

-
- _____

What I Learned Today:

-
- _____

Dreams:

-
- _____

Goals for Tomorrow:

-
- _____

Quote of the Day:

- _____

Day 99:

Date: _____
Mood: _____

Gratitude:

-
-
- _____

Today's Highlights:

-
- _____

Challenges or Struggles:

-
- _____

What I Learned Today:

-
- _____

Dreams:

-
- _____

Goals for Tomorrow:

-
- _____

Quote of the Day:

- _____

Day 100:

Date: _____

Mood: _____

Gratitude:

-
-
-    _____

Today's Highlights:

-
-    _____

Challenges or Struggles:

-
-    _____

What I Learned Today:

-
-    _____

Dreams:

-
-    _____

Goals for Tomorrow:

-
-    _____

Quote of the Day:

-    _____

Day 101:

Date: _____

Mood: _____

Gratitude:

-
-
- _____

Today's Highlights:

-
- _____

Challenges or Struggles:

-
- _____

What I Learned Today:

-
- _____

Dreams:

-
- _____

Goals for Tomorrow:

-
- _____

Quote of the Day:

- _____

Day 102:

Date: _____

Mood: _____

Gratitude:

-
-
-     _____

Today's Highlights:

-
-     _____

Challenges or Struggles:

-
-     _____

What I Learned Today:

-
-     _____

Dreams:

-
-     _____

Goals for Tomorrow:

-
-     _____

Quote of the Day:

-     _____

Day 103:

Date: _____

Mood: _____

Gratitude:

-
-
- _____

Today's Highlights:

-
- _____

Challenges or Struggles:

-
- _____

What I Learned Today:

-
- _____

Dreams:

-
- _____

Goals for Tomorrow:

-
- _____

Quote of the Day:

- _____

Day 104:

Date: _____

Mood: _____

Gratitude:

-
-
- _____

Today's Highlights:

-
- _____

Challenges or Struggles:

-
- _____

What I Learned Today:

-
- _____

Dreams:

-
- _____

Goals for Tomorrow:

-
- _____

Quote of the Day:

- _____

Day 105:

Date: _____

Mood: _____

Gratitude:

-
-
- _____

Today's Highlights:

-
- _____

Challenges or Struggles:

-
- _____

What I Learned Today:

-
- _____

Dreams:

-
- _____

Goals for Tomorrow:

-
- _____

Quote of the Day:

- _____

Day 106:

Date: _____

Mood: _____

Gratitude:

-
-
-   _____

Today's Highlights:

-
-   _____

Challenges or Struggles:

-
-   _____

What I Learned Today:

-
-   _____

Dreams:

-
-   _____

Goals for Tomorrow:

-
-   _____

Quote of the Day:

-   _____

Day 107:

Date: _____

Mood: _____

Gratitude:

-
-
- _____

Today's Highlights:

-
- _____

Challenges or Struggles:

-
- _____

What I Learned Today:

-
- _____

Dreams:

-
- _____

Goals for Tomorrow:

-
- _____

Quote of the Day:

- _____

Day 108:

Date: _____

Mood: _____

Gratitude:

-
-
- _____

Today's Highlights:

-
- _____

Challenges or Struggles:

-
- _____

What I Learned Today:

-
- _____

Dreams:

-
- _____

Goals for Tomorrow:

-
- _____

Quote of the Day:

- _____

Day 109:

Date: _____

Mood: _____

Gratitude:

-
-
-    _____

Today's Highlights:

-
-    _____

Challenges or Struggles:

-
-    _____

What I Learned Today:

-
-    _____

Dreams:

-
-    _____

Goals for Tomorrow:

-
-    _____

Quote of the Day:

-    _____

Day 110:

Date: _____

Mood: _____

Gratitude:

-
-
-    _____

Today's Highlights:

-
-    _____

Challenges or Struggles:

-
-    _____

What I Learned Today:

-
-    _____

Dreams:

-
-    _____

Goals for Tomorrow:

-
-    _____

Quote of the Day:

-    _____

Day 111:

Date: _____

Mood: _____

Gratitude:

-
-
- _____

Today's Highlights:

-
- _____

Challenges or Struggles:

-
- _____

What I Learned Today:

-
- _____

Dreams:

-
- _____

Goals for Tomorrow:

-
- _____

Quote of the Day:

- _____

Day 112:

Date: _____

Mood: _____

Gratitude:

-
-
- _____

Today's Highlights:

-
- _____

Challenges or Struggles:

-
- _____

What I Learned Today:

-
- _____

Dreams:

-
- _____

Goals for Tomorrow:

-
- _____

Quote of the Day:

- _____

Day 113:

Date: _____

Mood: _____

Gratitude:

-
-
- _____

Today's Highlights:

-
- _____

Challenges or Struggles:

-
- _____

What I Learned Today:

-
- _____

Dreams:

-
- _____

Goals for Tomorrow:

-
- _____

Quote of the Day:

- _____

Day 114:

Date: _____

Mood: _____

Gratitude:

- •
- •
- • _____

Today's Highlights:

- •
- • _____

Challenges or Struggles:

- •
- • _____

What I Learned Today:

- •
- • _____

Dreams:

- •
- • _____

Goals for Tomorrow:

- •
- • _____

Quote of the Day:

- • _____

Day 115:

Date: _____

Mood: _____

Gratitude:

-
-
- _____

Today's Highlights:

-
- _____

Challenges or Struggles:

-
- _____

What I Learned Today:

-
- _____

Dreams:

-
- _____

Goals for Tomorrow:

-
- _____

Quote of the Day:

- _____

Day 116:

Date: _____

Mood: _____

Gratitude:

-
-
- _____

Today's Highlights:

-
- _____

Challenges or Struggles:

-
- _____

What I Learned Today:

-
- _____

Dreams:

-
- _____

Goals for Tomorrow:

-
- _____

Quote of the Day:

- _____

Day 117:

Date: _____

Mood: _____

Gratitude:

-
-
- _____

Today's Highlights:

-
- _____

Challenges or Struggles:

-
- _____

What I Learned Today:

-
- _____

Dreams:

-
- _____

Goals for Tomorrow:

-
- _____

Quote of the Day:

- _____

Day 118:

Date: _____

Mood: _____

Gratitude:

-
-
- _____

Today's Highlights:

-
- _____

Challenges or Struggles:

-
- _____

What I Learned Today:

-
- _____

Dreams:

-
- _____

Goals for Tomorrow:

-
- _____

Quote of the Day:

- _____

Day 119:

Date: _____
Mood: _____

Gratitude:

-
-
- _____

Today's Highlights:

-
- _____

Challenges or Struggles:

-
- _____

What I Learned Today:

-
- _____

Dreams:

-
- _____

Goals for Tomorrow:

-
- _____

Quote of the Day:

- _____

Day 120:

Date: _____

Mood: _____

Gratitude:

-
-
- _____

Today's Highlights:

-
- _____

Challenges or Struggles:

-
- _____

What I Learned Today:

-
- _____

Dreams:

-
- _____

Goals for Tomorrow:

-
- _____

Quote of the Day:

- _____

Day 121:

Date: _____

Mood: _____

Gratitude:

-
-
- _____

Today's Highlights:

-
- _____

Challenges or Struggles:

-
- _____

What I Learned Today:

-
- _____

Dreams:

-
- _____

Goals for Tomorrow:

-
- _____

Quote of the Day:

- _____

Day 122:

Date: _____

Mood: _____

Gratitude:

-
-
- _____

Today's Highlights:

-
- _____

Challenges or Struggles:

-
- _____

What I Learned Today:

-
- _____

Dreams:

-
- _____

Goals for Tomorrow:

-
- _____

Quote of the Day:

- _____

Day 123:

Date: _____

Mood: _____

Gratitude:

-
-
-    _____

Today's Highlights:

-
-    _____

Challenges or Struggles:

-
-    _____

What I Learned Today:

-
-    _____

Dreams:

-
-    _____

Goals for Tomorrow:

-
-    _____

Quote of the Day:

-    _____

Day 124:

Date: _____

Mood: _____

Gratitude:

-
-
- _____

Today's Highlights:

-
- _____

Challenges or Struggles:

-
- _____

What I Learned Today:

-
- _____

Dreams:

-
- _____

Goals for Tomorrow:

-
- _____

Quote of the Day:

- _____

Day 125:

Date: _____

Mood: _____

Gratitude:

-
-
- _____

Today's Highlights:

-
- _____

Challenges or Struggles:

-
- _____

What I Learned Today:

-
- _____

Dreams:

-
- _____

Goals for Tomorrow:

-
- _____

Quote of the Day:

- _____

Day 126:

Date: _____

Mood: _____

Gratitude:

-
-
-   _____

Today's Highlights:

-
-   _____

Challenges or Struggles:

-
-   _____

What I Learned Today:

-
-   _____

Dreams:

-
-   _____

Goals for Tomorrow:

-
-   _____

Quote of the Day:

-   _____
-

Day 127:

Date: _____

Mood: _____

Gratitude:

-
-
- _____

Today's Highlights:

-
- _____

Challenges or Struggles:

-
- _____

What I Learned Today:

-
- _____

Dreams:

-
- _____

Goals for Tomorrow:

-
- _____

Quote of the Day:

- _____

Day 128:

Date: _____

Mood: _____

Gratitude:

-
-
- _____

Today's Highlights:

-
- _____

Challenges or Struggles:

-
- _____

What I Learned Today:

-
- _____

Dreams:

-
- _____

Goals for Tomorrow:

-
- _____

Quote of the Day:

- _____

Day 129:

Date: _____

Mood: _____

Gratitude:

-
-
- _____

Today's Highlights:

-
- _____

Challenges or Struggles:

-
- _____

What I Learned Today:

-
- _____

Dreams:

-
- _____

Goals for Tomorrow:

-
- _____

Quote of the Day:

- _____

Day 130:

Date: _____

Mood: _____

Gratitude:

-
-
- _____

Today's Highlights:

-
- _____

Challenges or Struggles:

-
- _____

What I Learned Today:

-
- _____

Dreams:

-
- _____

Goals for Tomorrow:

-
- _____

Quote of the Day:

- _____

Day 131:

Date: _____

Mood: _____

Gratitude:

-
-
- _____

Today's Highlights:

-
- _____

Challenges or Struggles:

-
- _____

What I Learned Today:

-
- _____

Dreams:

-
- _____

Goals for Tomorrow:

-
- _____

Quote of the Day:

- _____

Day 132:

Date: _____

Mood: _____

Gratitude:

-
-
- _____

Today's Highlights:

-
- _____

Challenges or Struggles:

-
- _____

What I Learned Today:

-
- _____

Dreams:

-
- _____

Goals for Tomorrow:

-
- _____

Quote of the Day:

- _____

Day 133:

Date: _____

Mood: _____

Gratitude:

-
-
- _____

Today's Highlights:

-
- _____

Challenges or Struggles:

-
- _____

What I Learned Today:

-
- _____

Dreams:

-
- _____

Goals for Tomorrow:

-
- _____

Quote of the Day:

- _____

Day 134:

Date: _____

Mood: _____

Gratitude:

-
-
-     _____

Today's Highlights:

-
-     _____

Challenges or Struggles:

-
-     _____

What I Learned Today:

-
-     _____

Dreams:

-
-     _____

Goals for Tomorrow:

-
-     _____

Quote of the Day:

-     _____

Day 135:

Date: _____

Mood: _____

Gratitude:

-
-
- _____

Today's Highlights:

-
- _____

Challenges or Struggles:

-
- _____

What I Learned Today:

-
- _____

Dreams:

-
- _____

Goals for Tomorrow:

-
- _____

Quote of the Day:

- _____

Day 136:

Date: _____

Mood: _____

Gratitude:

-
-
- _____

Today's Highlights:

-
- _____

Challenges or Struggles:

-
- _____

What I Learned Today:

-
- _____

Dreams:

-
- _____

Goals for Tomorrow:

-
- _____

Quote of the Day:

- _____

Day 137:

Date: _____

Mood: _____

Gratitude:

-
-
- _____

Today's Highlights:

-
- _____

Challenges or Struggles:

-
- _____

What I Learned Today:

-
- _____

Dreams:

-
- _____

Goals for Tomorrow:

-
- _____

Quote of the Day:

- _____

Day 138:

Date: _____

Mood: _____

Gratitude:

-
-
-     _____

Today's Highlights:

-
-     _____

Challenges or Struggles:

-
-     _____

What I Learned Today:

-
-     _____

Dreams:

-
-     _____

Goals for Tomorrow:

-
-     _____

Quote of the Day:

-     _____

Day 139:

Date: _____

Mood: _____

Gratitude:

-
-
- _____

Today's Highlights:

-
- _____

Challenges or Struggles:

-
- _____

What I Learned Today:

-
- _____

Dreams:

-
- _____

Goals for Tomorrow:

-
- _____

Quote of the Day:

- _____

Day 140:

Date: _____

Mood: _____

Gratitude:

-
-
- _____

Today's Highlights:

-
- _____

Challenges or Struggles:

-
- _____

What I Learned Today:

-
- _____

Dreams:

-
- _____

Goals for Tomorrow:

-
- _____

Quote of the Day:

- _____

Day 141:

Date: _____

Mood: _____

Gratitude:

-
-
- _____

Today's Highlights:

-
- _____

Challenges or Struggles:

-
- _____

What I Learned Today:

-
- _____

Dreams:

-
- _____

Goals for Tomorrow:

-
- _____

Quote of the Day:

- _____

Day 142:

Date: _____

Mood: _____

Gratitude:

-
-
- _____

Today's Highlights:

-
- _____

Challenges or Struggles:

-
- _____

What I Learned Today:

-
- _____

Dreams:

-
- _____

Goals for Tomorrow:

-
- _____

Quote of the Day:

- _____

Day 143:

Date: _____

Mood: _____

Gratitude:

-
-
- _____

Today's Highlights:

-
- _____

Challenges or Struggles:

-
- _____

What I Learned Today:

-
- _____

Dreams:

-
- _____

Goals for Tomorrow:

-
- _____

Quote of the Day:

- _____

Day 144:

Date: _____

Mood: _____

Gratitude:

-
-
- _____

Today's Highlights:

-
- _____

Challenges or Struggles:

-
- _____

What I Learned Today:

-
- _____

Dreams:

-
- _____

Goals for Tomorrow:

-
- _____

Quote of the Day:

- _____

Day 145:

Date: _____

Mood: _____

Gratitude:

-
-
-    _____

Today's Highlights:

-
-    _____

Challenges or Struggles:

-
-    _____

What I Learned Today:

-
-    _____

Dreams:

-
-    _____

Goals for Tomorrow:

-
-    _____

Quote of the Day:

-    _____

Day 146:

Date: _____

Mood: _____

Gratitude:

-
-
- _____

Today's Highlights:

-
- _____

Challenges or Struggles:

-
- _____

What I Learned Today:

-
- _____

Dreams:

-
- _____

Goals for Tomorrow:

-
- _____

Quote of the Day:

- _____

Day 147:

Date: _____

Mood: _____

Gratitude:

-
-
-     _____

Today's Highlights:

-
-     _____

Challenges or Struggles:

-
-     _____

What I Learned Today:

-
-     _____

Dreams:

-
-     _____

Goals for Tomorrow:

-
-     _____

Quote of the Day:

-     _____

Day 148:

Date: _____

Mood: _____

Gratitude:

-
-
- _____

Today's Highlights:

-
- _____

Challenges or Struggles:

-
- _____

What I Learned Today:

-
- _____

Dreams:

-
- _____

Goals for Tomorrow:

-
- _____

Quote of the Day:

- _____

Day 149:

Date: _____

Mood: _____

Gratitude:

-
-
- _____

Today's Highlights:

-
- _____

Challenges or Struggles:

-
- _____

What I Learned Today:

-
- _____

Dreams:

-
- _____

Goals for Tomorrow:

-
- _____

Quote of the Day:

- _____

Day 150:

Date: _____

Mood: _____

Gratitude:

-
-
- _____

Today's Highlights:

-
- _____

Challenges or Struggles:

-
- _____

What I Learned Today:

-
- _____

Dreams:

-
- _____

Goals for Tomorrow:

-
- _____

Quote of the Day:

- _____

Day 151:

Date: _____

Mood: _____

Gratitude:

-
-
- _____

Today's Highlights:

-
- _____

Challenges or Struggles:

-
- _____

What I Learned Today:

-
- _____

Dreams:

-
- _____

Goals for Tomorrow:

-
- _____

Quote of the Day:

- _____

Day 152:

Date: _____

Mood: _____

Gratitude:

-
-
- _____

Today's Highlights:

-
- _____

Challenges or Struggles:

-
- _____

What I Learned Today:

-
- _____

Dreams:

-
- _____

Goals for Tomorrow:

-
- _____

Quote of the Day:

- _____

Day 153:

Date: _____

Mood: _____

Gratitude:

-
-
- _____

Today's Highlights:

-
- _____

Challenges or Struggles:

-
- _____

What I Learned Today:

-
- _____

Dreams:

-
- _____

Goals for Tomorrow:

-
- _____

Quote of the Day:

- _____

Day 154:

Date: _____

Mood: _____

Gratitude:

-
-
- _____

Today's Highlights:

-
- _____

Challenges or Struggles:

-
- _____

What I Learned Today:

-
- _____

Dreams:

-
- _____

Goals for Tomorrow:

-
- _____

Quote of the Day:

- _____

Day 155:

Date: _____

Mood: _____

Gratitude:

-
-
- _____

Today's Highlights:

-
- _____

Challenges or Struggles:

-
- _____

What I Learned Today:

-
- _____

Dreams:

-
- _____

Goals for Tomorrow:

-
- _____

Quote of the Day:

- _____

Day 156:

Date: _____

Mood: _____

Gratitude:

-
-
-    _____

Today's Highlights:

-
-    _____

Challenges or Struggles:

-
-    _____

What I Learned Today:

-
-    _____

Dreams:

-
-    _____

Goals for Tomorrow:

-
-    _____

Quote of the Day:

-    _____

Day 157:

Date: _____

Mood: _____

Gratitude:

-
-
- _____

Today's Highlights:

-
- _____

Challenges or Struggles:

-
- _____

What I Learned Today:

-
- _____

Dreams:

-
- _____

Goals for Tomorrow:

-
- _____

Quote of the Day:

- _____

Day 158:

Date: _____

Mood: _____

Gratitude:

-
-
- _____

Today's Highlights:

-
- _____

Challenges or Struggles:

-
- _____

What I Learned Today:

-
- _____

Dreams:

-
- _____

Goals for Tomorrow:

-
- _____

Quote of the Day:

- _____

Day 159:

Date: _____

Mood: _____

Gratitude:

-
-
- _____

Today's Highlights:

-
- _____

Challenges or Struggles:

-
- _____

What I Learned Today:

-
- _____

Dreams:

-
- _____

Goals for Tomorrow:

-
- _____

Quote of the Day:

- _____

Day 160:

Date: _____

Mood: _____

Gratitude:

-
-
- _____

Today's Highlights:

-
- _____

Challenges or Struggles:

-
- _____

What I Learned Today:

-
- _____

Dreams:

-
- _____

Goals for Tomorrow:

-
- _____

Quote of the Day:

- _____

Day 161:

Date: _____

Mood: _____

Gratitude:

-
-
- _____

Today's Highlights:

-
- _____

Challenges or Struggles:

-
- _____

What I Learned Today:

-
- _____

Dreams:

-
- _____

Goals for Tomorrow:

-
- _____

Quote of the Day:

- _____

Day 162:

Date: _____

Mood: _____

Gratitude:

-
-
- _____

Today's Highlights:

-
- _____

Challenges or Struggles:

-
- _____

What I Learned Today:

-
- _____

Dreams:

-
- _____

Goals for Tomorrow:

-
- _____

Quote of the Day:

- _____
-

Day 163:

Date: _____

Mood: _____

Gratitude:

-
-
- _____

Today's Highlights:

-
- _____

Challenges or Struggles:

-
- _____

What I Learned Today:

-
- _____

Dreams:

-
- _____

Goals for Tomorrow:

-
- _____

Quote of the Day:

- _____

Day 164:

Date: _____

Mood: _____

Gratitude:

-
-
- _____

Today's Highlights:

-
- _____

Challenges or Struggles:

-
- _____

What I Learned Today:

-
- _____

Dreams:

-
- _____

Goals for Tomorrow:

-
- _____

Quote of the Day:

- _____

Day 165:

Date: _____

Mood: _____

Gratitude:

-
-
-     _____

Today's Highlights:

-
-     _____

Challenges or Struggles:

-
-     _____

What I Learned Today:

-
-     _____

Dreams:

-
-     _____

Goals for Tomorrow:

-
-     _____

Quote of the Day:

-     _____

Day 166:

Date: _____

Mood: _____

Gratitude:

-
-
-    _____

Today's Highlights:

-
-    _____

Challenges or Struggles:

-
-    _____

What I Learned Today:

-
-    _____

Dreams:

-
-    _____

Goals for Tomorrow:

-
-    _____

Quote of the Day:

-    _____

Day 167:

Date: _____

Mood: _____

Gratitude:

-
-
- _____

Today's Highlights:

-
- _____

Challenges or Struggles:

-
- _____

What I Learned Today:

-
- _____

Dreams:

-
- _____

Goals for Tomorrow:

-
- _____

Quote of the Day:

- _____

Day 168:

Date: _____

Mood: _____

Gratitude:

-
-
- _____

Today's Highlights:

-
- _____

Challenges or Struggles:

-
- _____

What I Learned Today:

-
- _____

Dreams:

-
- _____

Goals for Tomorrow:

-
- _____

Quote of the Day:

- _____

Day 169:

Date: _____

Mood: _____

Gratitude:

-
-
- _____

Today's Highlights:

-
- _____

Challenges or Struggles:

-
- _____

What I Learned Today:

-
- _____

Dreams:

-
- _____

Goals for Tomorrow:

-
- _____

Quote of the Day:

- _____

Day 170:

Date: _____

Mood: _____

Gratitude:

-
-
-     _____

Today's Highlights:

-
-     _____

Challenges or Struggles:

-
-     _____

What I Learned Today:

-
-     _____

Dreams:

-
-     _____

Goals for Tomorrow:

-
-     _____

Quote of the Day:

-     _____

Day 171:

Date: _____

Mood: _____

Gratitude:

-
-
- _____

Today's Highlights:

-
- _____

Challenges or Struggles:

-
- _____

What I Learned Today:

-
- _____

Dreams:

-
- _____

Goals for Tomorrow:

-
- _____

Quote of the Day:

- _____

Day 172:

Date: _____

Mood: _____

Gratitude:

-
-
- _____

Today's Highlights:

-
- _____

Challenges or Struggles:

-
- _____

What I Learned Today:

-
- _____

Dreams:

-
- _____

Goals for Tomorrow:

-
- _____

Quote of the Day:

- _____

Day 173:

Date: _____

Mood: _____

Gratitude:

-
-
- _____

Today's Highlights:

-
- _____

Challenges or Struggles:

-
- _____

What I Learned Today:

-
- _____

Dreams:

-
- _____

Goals for Tomorrow:

-
- _____

Quote of the Day:

- _____

Day 174:

Date: _____

Mood: _____

Gratitude:

-
-
-   _____

Today's Highlights:

-
-   _____

Challenges or Struggles:

-
-   _____

What I Learned Today:

-
-   _____

Dreams:

-
-   _____

Goals for Tomorrow:

-
-   _____

Quote of the Day:

-   _____

Day 175:

Date: _____

Mood: _____

Gratitude:

-
-
- _____

Today's Highlights:

-
- _____

Challenges or Struggles:

-
- _____

What I Learned Today:

-
- _____

Dreams:

-
- _____

Goals for Tomorrow:

-
- _____

Quote of the Day:

- _____

Day 176:

Date: _____

Mood: _____

Gratitude:

-
-
- _____

Today's Highlights:

-
- _____

Challenges or Struggles:

-
- _____

What I Learned Today:

-
- _____

Dreams:

-
- _____

Goals for Tomorrow:

-
- _____

Quote of the Day:

- _____

Day 177:

Date: _____

Mood: _____

Gratitude:

-
-
- _____

Today's Highlights:

-
- _____

Challenges or Struggles:

-
- _____

What I Learned Today:

-
- _____

Dreams:

-
- _____

Goals for Tomorrow:

-
- _____

Quote of the Day:

- _____

Day 178:

Date: _____

Mood: _____

Gratitude:

-
-
- _____

Today's Highlights:

-
- _____

Challenges or Struggles:

-
- _____

What I Learned Today:

-
- _____

Dreams:

-
- _____

Goals for Tomorrow:

-
- _____

Quote of the Day:

- _____

Day 179:

Date: _____
Mood: _____

Gratitude:

-
-
- _____

Today's Highlights:

-
- _____

Challenges or Struggles:

-
- _____

What I Learned Today:

-
- _____

Dreams:

-
- _____

Goals for Tomorrow:

-
- _____

Quote of the Day:

- _____

Day 180:

Date: _____

Mood: _____

Gratitude:

-
-
-   _____

Today's Highlights:

-
-   _____

Challenges or Struggles:

-
-   _____

What I Learned Today:

-
-   _____

Dreams:

-
-   _____

Goals for Tomorrow:

-
-   _____

Quote of the Day:

-   _____

Day 181:

Date: _____

Mood: _____

Gratitude:

-
-
- _____

Today's Highlights:

-
- _____

Challenges or Struggles:

-
- _____

What I Learned Today:

-
- _____

Dreams:

-
- _____

Goals for Tomorrow:

-
- _____

Quote of the Day:

- _____

Day 182:

Date: _____

Mood: _____

Gratitude:

-
-
- _____

Today's Highlights:

-
- _____

Challenges or Struggles:

-
- _____

What I Learned Today:

-
- _____

Dreams:

-
- _____

Goals for Tomorrow:

-
- _____

Quote of the Day:

- _____

Day 183:

Date: _____

Mood: _____

Gratitude:

-
-
- _____

Today's Highlights:

-
- _____

Challenges or Struggles:

-
- _____

What I Learned Today:

-
- _____

Dreams:

-
- _____

Goals for Tomorrow:

-
- _____

Quote of the Day:

- _____

Day 184:

Date: _____

Mood: _____

Gratitude:

-
-
- _____

Today's Highlights:

-
- _____

Challenges or Struggles:

-
- _____

What I Learned Today:

-
- _____

Dreams:

-
- _____

Goals for Tomorrow:

-
- _____

Quote of the Day:

- _____

Day 185:

Date: _____

Mood: _____

Gratitude:

-
-
- _____

Today's Highlights:

-
- _____

Challenges or Struggles:

-
- _____

What I Learned Today:

-
- _____

Dreams:

-
- _____

Goals for Tomorrow:

-
- _____

Quote of the Day:

- _____

Day 186:

Date: _____

Mood: _____

Gratitude:

-
-
-          _____

Today's Highlights:

-
-          _____

Challenges or Struggles:

-
-          _____

What I Learned Today:

-
-          _____

Dreams:

-
-          _____

Goals for Tomorrow:

-
-          _____

Quote of the Day:

-          _____

Day 187:

Date: _____

Mood: _____

Gratitude:

-
-
- _____

Today's Highlights:

-
- _____

Challenges or Struggles:

-
- _____

What I Learned Today:

-
- _____

Dreams:

-
- _____

Goals for Tomorrow:

-
- _____

Quote of the Day:

- _____

Day 188:

Date: _____

Mood: _____

Gratitude:

-
-
-     _____

Today's Highlights:

-
-     _____

Challenges or Struggles:

-
-     _____

What I Learned Today:

-
-     _____

Dreams:

-
-     _____

Goals for Tomorrow:

-
-     _____

Quote of the Day:

-     _____

Day 189:

Date: _____

Mood: _____

Gratitude:

-
-
- _____

Today's Highlights:

-
- _____

Challenges or Struggles:

-
- _____

What I Learned Today:

-
- _____

Dreams:

-
- _____

Goals for Tomorrow:

-
- _____

Quote of the Day:

- _____

Day 190:

Date: _____

Mood: _____

Gratitude:

-
-
- _____

Today's Highlights:

-
- _____

Challenges or Struggles:

-
- _____

What I Learned Today:

-
- _____

Dreams:

-
- _____

Goals for Tomorrow:

-
- _____

Quote of the Day:

- _____

Day 191:

Date: _____

Mood: _____

Gratitude:

-
-
- _____

Today's Highlights:

-
- _____

Challenges or Struggles:

-
- _____

What I Learned Today:

-
- _____

Dreams:

-
- _____

Goals for Tomorrow:

-
- _____

Quote of the Day:

- _____

Day 192:

Date: _____

Mood: _____

Gratitude:

-
-
- _____

Today's Highlights:

-
- _____

Challenges or Struggles:

-
- _____

What I Learned Today:

-
- _____

Dreams:

-
- _____

Goals for Tomorrow:

-
- _____

Quote of the Day:

- _____

Day 193:

Date: _____

Mood: _____

Gratitude:

-
-
- _____

Today's Highlights:

-
- _____

Challenges or Struggles:

-
- _____

What I Learned Today:

-
- _____

Dreams:

-
- _____

Goals for Tomorrow:

-
- _____

Quote of the Day:

- _____

Day 194:

Date: _____

Mood: _____

Gratitude:

-
-
- _____

Today's Highlights:

-
- _____

Challenges or Struggles:

-
- _____

What I Learned Today:

-
- _____

Dreams:

-
- _____

Goals for Tomorrow:

-
- _____

Quote of the Day:

- _____

Day 195:

Date: _____

Mood: _____

Gratitude:

-
-
- _____

Today's Highlights:

-
- _____

Challenges or Struggles:

-
- _____

What I Learned Today:

-
- _____

Dreams:

-
- _____

Goals for Tomorrow:

-
- _____

Quote of the Day:

- _____

Day 196:

Date: _____
Mood: _____

Gratitude:

-
-
- _____

Today's Highlights:

-
- _____

Challenges or Struggles:

-
- _____

What I Learned Today:

-
- _____

Dreams:

-
- _____

Goals for Tomorrow:

-
- _____

Quote of the Day:

- _____

Day 197:

Date: _____

Mood: _____

Gratitude:

-
-
- _____

Today's Highlights:

-
- _____

Challenges or Struggles:

-
- _____

What I Learned Today:

-
- _____

Dreams:

-
- _____

Goals for Tomorrow:

-
- _____

Quote of the Day:

- _____

Day 198:

Date: _____

Mood: _____

Gratitude:

-
-
- _____

Today's Highlights:

-
- _____

Challenges or Struggles:

-
- _____

What I Learned Today:

-
- _____

Dreams:

-
- _____

Goals for Tomorrow:

-
- _____

Quote of the Day:

- _____
-

Day 199:

Date: _____

Mood: _____

Gratitude:

-
-
- _____

Today's Highlights:

-
- _____

Challenges or Struggles:

-
- _____

What I Learned Today:

-
- _____

Dreams:

-
- _____

Goals for Tomorrow:

-
- _____

Quote of the Day:

- _____

Day 200:

Date: _____

Mood: _____

Gratitude:

-
-
- _____

Today's Highlights:

-
- _____

Challenges or Struggles:

-
- _____

What I Learned Today:

-
- _____

Dreams:

-
- _____

Goals for Tomorrow:

-
- _____

Quote of the Day:

- _____

Day 201:

Date: _____

Mood: _____

Gratitude:

-
-
- _____

Today's Highlights:

-
- _____

Challenges or Struggles:

-
- _____

What I Learned Today:

-
- _____

Dreams:

-
- _____

Goals for Tomorrow:

-
- _____

Quote of the Day:

- _____

Day 202:

Date: _____

Mood: _____

Gratitude:

-
-
-    _____

Today's Highlights:

-
-    _____

Challenges or Struggles:

-
-    _____

What I Learned Today:

-
-    _____

Dreams:

-
-    _____

Goals for Tomorrow:

-
-    _____

Quote of the Day:

-    _____

Day 203:

Date: _____

Mood: _____

Gratitude:

-
-
- _____

Today's Highlights:

-
- _____

Challenges or Struggles:

-
- _____

What I Learned Today:

-
- _____

Dreams:

-
- _____

Goals for Tomorrow:

-
- _____

Quote of the Day:

- _____

Day 204:

Date: _____

Mood: _____

Gratitude:

-
-
- _____

Today's Highlights:

-
- _____

Challenges or Struggles:

-
- _____

What I Learned Today:

-
- _____

Dreams:

-
- _____

Goals for Tomorrow:

-
- _____

Quote of the Day:

- _____

Day 205:

Date: _____

Mood: _____

Gratitude:

-
-
- _____

Today's Highlights:

-
- _____

Challenges or Struggles:

-
- _____

What I Learned Today:

-
- _____

Dreams:

-
- _____

Goals for Tomorrow:

-
- _____

Quote of the Day:

- _____

Day 206:

Date: _____

Mood: _____

Gratitude:

-
-
- _____

Today's Highlights:

-
- _____

Challenges or Struggles:

-
- _____

What I Learned Today:

-
- _____

Dreams:

-
- _____

Goals for Tomorrow:

-
- _____

Quote of the Day:

- _____

Day 207:

Date: _____

Mood: _____

Gratitude:

-
-
- _____

Today's Highlights:

-
- _____

Challenges or Struggles:

-
- _____

What I Learned Today:

-
- _____

Dreams:

-
- _____

Goals for Tomorrow:

-
- _____

Quote of the Day:

- _____

Day 208:

Date: _____

Mood: _____

Gratitude:

-
-
- _____

Today's Highlights:

-
- _____

Challenges or Struggles:

-
- _____

What I Learned Today:

-
- _____

Dreams:

-
- _____

Goals for Tomorrow:

-
- _____

Quote of the Day:

- _____

Day 209:

Date: _____

Mood: _____

Gratitude:

-
-
- _____

Today's Highlights:

-
- _____

Challenges or Struggles:

-
- _____

What I Learned Today:

-
- _____

Dreams:

-
- _____

Goals for Tomorrow:

-
- _____

Quote of the Day:

- _____

Day 210:

Date: _____

Mood: _____

Gratitude:

-
-
- _____

Today's Highlights:

-
- _____

Challenges or Struggles:

-
- _____

What I Learned Today:

-
- _____

Dreams:

-
- _____

Goals for Tomorrow:

-
- _____

Quote of the Day:

- _____

Day 211:

Date: _____

Mood: _____

Gratitude:

-
-
- _____

Today's Highlights:

-
- _____

Challenges or Struggles:

-
- _____

What I Learned Today:

-
- _____

Dreams:

-
- _____

Goals for Tomorrow:

-
- _____

Quote of the Day:

- _____

Day 212:

Date: _____

Mood: _____

Gratitude:

-
-
- _____

Today's Highlights:

-
- _____

Challenges or Struggles:

-
- _____

What I Learned Today:

-
- _____

Dreams:

-
- _____

Goals for Tomorrow:

-
- _____

Quote of the Day:

- _____

Day 213:

Date: _____

Mood: _____

Gratitude:

-
-
- _____

Today's Highlights:

-
- _____

Challenges or Struggles:

-
- _____

What I Learned Today:

-
- _____

Dreams:

-
- _____

Goals for Tomorrow:

-
- _____

Quote of the Day:

- _____

Day 214:

Date: _____

Mood: _____

Gratitude:

-
-
-     _____

Today's Highlights:

-
-     _____

Challenges or Struggles:

-
-     _____

What I Learned Today:

-
-     _____

Dreams:

-
-     _____

Goals for Tomorrow:

-
-     _____

Quote of the Day:

-     _____

Day 215:

Date: _____
Mood: _____

Gratitude:

-
-
- _____

Today's Highlights:

-
- _____

Challenges or Struggles:

-
- _____

What I Learned Today:

-
- _____

Dreams:

-
- _____

Goals for Tomorrow:

-
- _____

Quote of the Day:

- _____

Day 216:

Date: _____

Mood: _____

Gratitude:

-
-
- _____

Today's Highlights:

-
- _____

Challenges or Struggles:

-
- _____

What I Learned Today:

-
- _____

Dreams:

-
- _____

Goals for Tomorrow:

-
- _____

Quote of the Day:

- _____

Day 217:

Date: _____

Mood: _____

Gratitude:

-
-
-    _____

Today's Highlights:

-
-    _____

Challenges or Struggles:

-
-    _____

What I Learned Today:

-
-    _____

Dreams:

-
-    _____

Goals for Tomorrow:

-
-    _____

Quote of the Day:

-    _____

Day 218:

Date: _____

Mood: _____

Gratitude:

-
-
- _____

Today's Highlights:

-
- _____

Challenges or Struggles:

-
- _____

What I Learned Today:

-
- _____

Dreams:

-
- _____

Goals for Tomorrow:

-
- _____

Quote of the Day:

- _____

Day 219:

Date: _____

Mood: _____

Gratitude:

-
-
- _____

Today's Highlights:

-
- _____

Challenges or Struggles:

-
- _____

What I Learned Today:

-
- _____

Dreams:

-
- _____

Goals for Tomorrow:

-
- _____

Quote of the Day:

- _____

Day 220:

Date: _____

Mood: _____

Gratitude:

-
-
- _____

Today's Highlights:

-
- _____

Challenges or Struggles:

-
- _____

What I Learned Today:

-
- _____

Dreams:

-
- _____

Goals for Tomorrow:

-
- _____

Quote of the Day:

- _____

Day 221:

Date: _____

Mood: _____

Gratitude:

-
-
- _____

Today's Highlights:

-
- _____

Challenges or Struggles:

-
- _____

What I Learned Today:

-
- _____

Dreams:

-
- _____

Goals for Tomorrow:

-
- _____

Quote of the Day:

- _____

Day 222:

Date: _____

Mood: _____

Gratitude:

-
-
- _____

Today's Highlights:

-
- _____

Challenges or Struggles:

-
- _____

What I Learned Today:

-
- _____

Dreams:

-
- _____

Goals for Tomorrow:

-
- _____

Quote of the Day:

- _____

Day 223:

Date: _____

Mood: _____

Gratitude:

-
-
-   _____

Today's Highlights:

-
-   _____

Challenges or Struggles:

-
-   _____

What I Learned Today:

-
-   _____

Dreams:

-
-   _____

Goals for Tomorrow:

-
-   _____

Quote of the Day:

-   _____

Day 224:

Date: _____

Mood: _____

Gratitude:

-
-
-      _____

Today's Highlights:

-
-      _____

Challenges or Struggles:

-
-      _____

What I Learned Today:

-
-      _____

Dreams:

-
-      _____

Goals for Tomorrow:

-
-      _____

Quote of the Day:

-      _____

Day 225:

Date: _____

Mood: _____

Gratitude:

-
-
- _____

Today's Highlights:

-
- _____

Challenges or Struggles:

-
- _____

What I Learned Today:

-
- _____

Dreams:

-
- _____

Goals for Tomorrow:

-
- _____

Quote of the Day:

- _____

Day 226:

Date: _____

Mood: _____

Gratitude:

-
-
- _____

Today's Highlights:

-
- _____

Challenges or Struggles:

-
- _____

What I Learned Today:

-
- _____

Dreams:

-
- _____

Goals for Tomorrow:

-
- _____

Quote of the Day:

- _____

Day 227:

Date: _____

Mood: _____

Gratitude:

-
-
- _____

Today's Highlights:

-
- _____

Challenges or Struggles:

-
- _____

What I Learned Today:

-
- _____

Dreams:

-
- _____

Goals for Tomorrow:

-
- _____

Quote of the Day:

- _____

Day 228:

Date: _____

Mood: _____

Gratitude:

-
-
- _____

Today's Highlights:

-
- _____

Challenges or Struggles:

-
- _____

What I Learned Today:

-
- _____

Dreams:

-
- _____

Goals for Tomorrow:

-
- _____

Quote of the Day:

- _____

Day 229:

Date: _____

Mood: _____

Gratitude:

-
-
-   _____

Today's Highlights:

-
-   _____

Challenges or Struggles:

-
-   _____

What I Learned Today:

-
-   _____

Dreams:

-
-   _____

Goals for Tomorrow:

-
-   _____

Quote of the Day:

-   _____

Day 230:

Date: _____

Mood: _____

Gratitude:

-
-
- _____

Today's Highlights:

-
- _____

Challenges or Struggles:

-
- _____

What I Learned Today:

-
- _____

Dreams:

-
- _____

Goals for Tomorrow:

-
- _____

Quote of the Day:

- _____

Day 231:

Date: _____

Mood: _____

Gratitude:

-
-
- _____

Today's Highlights:

-
- _____

Challenges or Struggles:

-
- _____

What I Learned Today:

-
- _____

Dreams:

-
- _____

Goals for Tomorrow:

-
- _____

Quote of the Day:

- _____

Day 232:

Date: _____

Mood: _____

Gratitude:

-
-
- _____

Today's Highlights:

-
- _____

Challenges or Struggles:

-
- _____

What I Learned Today:

-
- _____

Dreams:

-
- _____

Goals for Tomorrow:

-
- _____

Quote of the Day:

- _____

Day 233:

Date: _____

Mood: _____

Gratitude:

-
-
- _____

Today's Highlights:

-
- _____

Challenges or Struggles:

-
- _____

What I Learned Today:

-
- _____

Dreams:

-
- _____

Goals for Tomorrow:

-
- _____

Quote of the Day:

- _____

Day 234:

Date: _____

Mood: _____

Gratitude:

-
-
-    _____

Today's Highlights:

-
-    _____

Challenges or Struggles:

-
-    _____

What I Learned Today:

-
-    _____

Dreams:

-
-    _____

Goals for Tomorrow:

-
-    _____

Quote of the Day:

-    _____
-

Day 235:

Date: _____

Mood: _____

Gratitude:

-
-
-     _____

Today's Highlights:

-
-     _____

Challenges or Struggles:

-
-     _____

What I Learned Today:

-
-     _____

Dreams:

-
-     _____

Goals for Tomorrow:

-
-     _____

Quote of the Day:

-     _____

Day 236:

Date: _____

Mood: _____

Gratitude:

-
-
- _____

Today's Highlights:

-
- _____

Challenges or Struggles:

-
- _____

What I Learned Today:

-
- _____

Dreams:

-
- _____

Goals for Tomorrow:

-
- _____

Quote of the Day:

- _____

Day 237:

Date: _____

Mood: _____

Gratitude:

-
-
-    _____

Today's Highlights:

-
-    _____

Challenges or Struggles:

-
-    _____

What I Learned Today:

-
-    _____

Dreams:

-
-    _____

Goals for Tomorrow:

-
-    _____

Quote of the Day:

-    _____

Day 238:

Date: _____

Mood: _____

Gratitude:

-
-
- _____

Today's Highlights:

-
- _____

Challenges or Struggles:

-
- _____

What I Learned Today:

-
- _____

Dreams:

-
- _____

Goals for Tomorrow:

-
- _____

Quote of the Day:

- _____

Day 239:

Date: _____

Mood: _____

Gratitude:

-
-
- _____

Today's Highlights:

-
- _____

Challenges or Struggles:

-
- _____

What I Learned Today:

-
- _____

Dreams:

-
- _____

Goals for Tomorrow:

-
- _____

Quote of the Day:

- _____

Day 240:

Date: _____

Mood: _____

Gratitude:

-
-
- _____

Today's Highlights:

-
- _____

Challenges or Struggles:

-
- _____

What I Learned Today:

-
- _____

Dreams:

-
- _____

Goals for Tomorrow:

-
- _____

Quote of the Day:

- _____

Day 241:

Date: _____

Mood: _____

Gratitude:

-
-
-   _____

Today's Highlights:

-
-   _____

Challenges or Struggles:

-
-   _____

What I Learned Today:

-
-   _____

Dreams:

-
-   _____

Goals for Tomorrow:

-
-   _____

Quote of the Day:

-   _____

Day 242:

Date: _____

Mood: _____

Gratitude:

-
-
- _____

Today's Highlights:

-
- _____

Challenges or Struggles:

-
- _____

What I Learned Today:

-
- _____

Dreams:

-
- _____

Goals for Tomorrow:

-
- _____

Quote of the Day:

- _____

Day 243:

Date: _____

Mood: _____

Gratitude:

-
-
- _____

Today's Highlights:

-
- _____

Challenges or Struggles:

-
- _____

What I Learned Today:

-
- _____

Dreams:

-
- _____

Goals for Tomorrow:

-
- _____

Quote of the Day:

- _____

Day 244:

Date: _____

Mood: _____

Gratitude:

-
-
- _____

Today's Highlights:

-
- _____

Challenges or Struggles:

-
- _____

What I Learned Today:

-
- _____

Dreams:

-
- _____

Goals for Tomorrow:

-
- _____

Quote of the Day:

- _____

Day 245:

Date: _____

Mood: _____

Gratitude:

-
-
- _____

Today's Highlights:

-
- _____

Challenges or Struggles:

-
- _____

What I Learned Today:

-
- _____

Dreams:

-
- _____

Goals for Tomorrow:

-
- _____

Quote of the Day:

- _____

Day 246:

Date: _____

Mood: _____

Gratitude:

-
-
-   _____

Today's Highlights:

-
-   _____

Challenges or Struggles:

-
-   _____

What I Learned Today:

-
-   _____

Dreams:

-
-   _____

Goals for Tomorrow:

-
-   _____

Quote of the Day:

-   _____

Day 247:

Date: _____

Mood: _____

Gratitude:

-
-
- _____

Today's Highlights:

-
- _____

Challenges or Struggles:

-
- _____

What I Learned Today:

-
- _____

Dreams:

-
- _____

Goals for Tomorrow:

-
- _____

Quote of the Day:

- _____

Day 248:

Date: _____

Mood: _____

Gratitude:

-
-
- _____

Today's Highlights:

-
- _____

Challenges or Struggles:

-
- _____

What I Learned Today:

-
- _____

Dreams:

-
- _____

Goals for Tomorrow:

-
- _____

Quote of the Day:

- _____

Day 249:

Date: _____

Mood: _____

Gratitude:

-
-
- _____

Today's Highlights:

-
- _____

Challenges or Struggles:

-
- _____

What I Learned Today:

-
- _____

Dreams:

-
- _____

Goals for Tomorrow:

-
- _____

Quote of the Day:

- _____

Day 250:

Date: _____

Mood: _____

Gratitude:

-
-
- _____

Today's Highlights:

-
- _____

Challenges or Struggles:

-
- _____

What I Learned Today:

-
- _____

Dreams:

-
- _____

Goals for Tomorrow:

-
- _____

Quote of the Day:

- _____

Day 251:

Date: _____

Mood: _____

Gratitude:

-
-
- _____

Today's Highlights:

-
- _____

Challenges or Struggles:

-
- _____

What I Learned Today:

-
- _____

Dreams:

-
- _____

Goals for Tomorrow:

-
- _____

Quote of the Day:

- _____

Day 252:

Date: _____

Mood: _____

Gratitude:

-
-
- _____

Today's Highlights:

-
- _____

Challenges or Struggles:

-
- _____

What I Learned Today:

-
- _____

Dreams:

-
- _____

Goals for Tomorrow:

-
- _____

Quote of the Day:

- _____

Day 253:

Date: _____

Mood: _____

Gratitude:

-
-
- _____

Today's Highlights:

-
- _____

Challenges or Struggles:

-
- _____

What I Learned Today:

-
- _____

Dreams:

-
- _____

Goals for Tomorrow:

-
- _____

Quote of the Day:

- _____

Day 254:

Date: _____

Mood: _____

Gratitude:

-
-
- _____

Today's Highlights:

-
- _____

Challenges or Struggles:

-
- _____

What I Learned Today:

-
- _____

Dreams:

-
- _____

Goals for Tomorrow:

-
- _____

Quote of the Day:

- _____

Day 255:

Date: _____

Mood: _____

Gratitude:

-
-
-    _____

Today's Highlights:

-
-    _____

Challenges or Struggles:

-
-    _____

What I Learned Today:

-
-    _____

Dreams:

-
-    _____

Goals for Tomorrow:

-
-    _____

Quote of the Day:

-    _____

Day 256:

Date: _____

Mood: _____

Gratitude:

-
-
- _____

Today's Highlights:

-
- _____

Challenges or Struggles:

-
- _____

What I Learned Today:

-
- _____

Dreams:

-
- _____

Goals for Tomorrow:

-
- _____

Quote of the Day:

- _____

Day 257:

Date: _____

Mood: _____

Gratitude:

-
-
- _____

Today's Highlights:

-
- _____

Challenges or Struggles:

-
- _____

What I Learned Today:

-
- _____

Dreams:

-
- _____

Goals for Tomorrow:

-
- _____

Quote of the Day:

- _____

Day 258:

Date: _____

Mood: _____

Gratitude:

-
-
- _____

Today's Highlights:

-
- _____

Challenges or Struggles:

-
- _____

What I Learned Today:

-
- _____

Dreams:

-
- _____

Goals for Tomorrow:

-
- _____

Quote of the Day:

- _____

Day 259:

Date: _____

Mood: _____

Gratitude:

-
-
- _____

Today's Highlights:

-
- _____

Challenges or Struggles:

-
- _____

What I Learned Today:

-
- _____

Dreams:

-
- _____

Goals for Tomorrow:

-
- _____

Quote of the Day:

- _____

Day 260:

Date: _____

Mood: _____

Gratitude:

-
-
-    _____

Today's Highlights:

-
-    _____

Challenges or Struggles:

-
-    _____

What I Learned Today:

-
-    _____

Dreams:

-
-    _____

Goals for Tomorrow:

-
-    _____

Quote of the Day:

-    _____

Day 261:

Date: _____

Mood: _____

Gratitude:

-
-
- _____

Today's Highlights:

-
- _____

Challenges or Struggles:

-
- _____

What I Learned Today:

-
- _____

Dreams:

-
- _____

Goals for Tomorrow:

-
- _____

Quote of the Day:

- _____

Day 262:

Date: _____

Mood: _____

Gratitude:

-
-
- _____

Today's Highlights:

-
- _____

Challenges or Struggles:

-
- _____

What I Learned Today:

-
- _____

Dreams:

-
- _____

Goals for Tomorrow:

-
- _____

Quote of the Day:

- _____

Day 263:

Date: _____

Mood: _____

Gratitude:

-
-
- _____

Today's Highlights:

-
- _____

Challenges or Struggles:

-
- _____

What I Learned Today:

-
- _____

Dreams:

-
- _____

Goals for Tomorrow:

-
- _____

Quote of the Day:

- _____

Day 264:

Date: _____

Mood: _____

Gratitude:

-
-
- _____

Today's Highlights:

-
- _____

Challenges or Struggles:

-
- _____

What I Learned Today:

-
- _____

Dreams:

-
- _____

Goals for Tomorrow:

-
- _____

Quote of the Day:

- _____

Day 265:

Date: _____

Mood: _____

Gratitude:

-
-
- _____

Today's Highlights:

-
- _____

Challenges or Struggles:

-
- _____

What I Learned Today:

-
- _____

Dreams:

-
- _____

Goals for Tomorrow:

-
- _____

Quote of the Day:

- _____

Day 266:

Date: _____

Mood: _____

Gratitude:

-
-
- _____

Today's Highlights:

-
- _____

Challenges or Struggles:

-
- _____

What I Learned Today:

-
- _____

Dreams:

-
- _____

Goals for Tomorrow:

-
- _____

Quote of the Day:

- _____

Day 267:

Date: _____

Mood: _____

Gratitude:

-
-
- _____

Today's Highlights:

-
- _____

Challenges or Struggles:

-
- _____

What I Learned Today:

-
- _____

Dreams:

-
- _____

Goals for Tomorrow:

-
- _____

Quote of the Day:

- _____

Day 268:

Date: _____

Mood: _____

Gratitude:

-
-
- _____

Today's Highlights:

-
- _____

Challenges or Struggles:

-
- _____

What I Learned Today:

-
- _____

Dreams:

-
- _____

Goals for Tomorrow:

-
- _____

Quote of the Day:

- _____

Day 269:

Date: _____

Mood: _____

Gratitude:

-
-
- _____

Today's Highlights:

-
- _____

Challenges or Struggles:

-
- _____

What I Learned Today:

-
- _____

Dreams:

-
- _____

Goals for Tomorrow:

-
- _____

Quote of the Day:

- _____

Day 270:

Date: _____

Mood: _____

Gratitude:

-
-
- _____

Today's Highlights:

-
- _____

Challenges or Struggles:

-
- _____

What I Learned Today:

-
- _____

Dreams:

-
- _____

Goals for Tomorrow:

-
- _____

Quote of the Day:

- _____
-

Day 271:

Date: _____

Mood: _____

Gratitude:

-
-
- _____

Today's Highlights:

-
- _____

Challenges or Struggles:

-
- _____

What I Learned Today:

-
- _____

Dreams:

-
- _____

Goals for Tomorrow:

-
- _____

Quote of the Day:

- _____

Day 272:

Date: _____

Mood: _____

Gratitude:

-
-
- _____

Today's Highlights:

-
- _____

Challenges or Struggles:

-
- _____

What I Learned Today:

-
- _____

Dreams:

-
- _____

Goals for Tomorrow:

-
- _____

Quote of the Day:

- _____

Day 273:

Date: _____

Mood: _____

Gratitude:

-
-
- _____

Today's Highlights:

-
- _____

Challenges or Struggles:

-
- _____

What I Learned Today:

-
- _____

Dreams:

-
- _____

Goals for Tomorrow:

-
- _____

Quote of the Day:

- _____

Day 274:

Date: _____

Mood: _____

Gratitude:

-
-
- _____

Today's Highlights:

-
- _____

Challenges or Struggles:

-
- _____

What I Learned Today:

-
- _____

Dreams:

-
- _____

Goals for Tomorrow:

-
- _____

Quote of the Day:

- _____

Day 275:

Date: _____

Mood: _____

Gratitude:

-
-
- _____

Today's Highlights:

-
- _____

Challenges or Struggles:

-
- _____

What I Learned Today:

-
- _____

Dreams:

-
- _____

Goals for Tomorrow:

-
- _____

Quote of the Day:

- _____

Day 276:

Date: _____

Mood: _____

Gratitude:

-
-
- _____

Today's Highlights:

-
- _____

Challenges or Struggles:

-
- _____

What I Learned Today:

-
- _____

Dreams:

-
- _____

Goals for Tomorrow:

-
- _____

Quote of the Day:

- _____

Day 277:

Date: _____

Mood: _____

Gratitude:

-
-
- _____

Today's Highlights:

-
- _____

Challenges or Struggles:

-
- _____

What I Learned Today:

-
- _____

Dreams:

-
- _____

Goals for Tomorrow:

-
- _____

Quote of the Day:

- _____

Day 278:

Date: _____

Mood: _____

Gratitude:

-
-
- _____

Today's Highlights:

-
- _____

Challenges or Struggles:

-
- _____

What I Learned Today:

-
- _____

Dreams:

-
- _____

Goals for Tomorrow:

-
- _____

Quote of the Day:

- _____

Day 279:

Date: _____

Mood: _____

Gratitude:

-
-
- _____

Today's Highlights:

-
- _____

Challenges or Struggles:

-
- _____

What I Learned Today:

-
- _____

Dreams:

-
- _____

Goals for Tomorrow:

-
- _____

Quote of the Day:

- _____

Day 280:

Date: _____

Mood: _____

Gratitude:

-
-
- _____

Today's Highlights:

-
- _____

Challenges or Struggles:

-
- _____

What I Learned Today:

-
- _____

Dreams:

-
- _____

Goals for Tomorrow:

-
- _____

Quote of the Day:

- _____

Day 281:

Date: _____

Mood: _____

Gratitude:

-
-
- _____

Today's Highlights:

-
- _____

Challenges or Struggles:

-
- _____

What I Learned Today:

-
- _____

Dreams:

-
- _____

Goals for Tomorrow:

-
- _____

Quote of the Day:

- _____

Day 282:

Date: _____

Mood: _____

Gratitude:

-
-
-     _____

Today's Highlights:

-
-     _____

Challenges or Struggles:

-
-     _____

What I Learned Today:

-
-     _____

Dreams:

-
-     _____

Goals for Tomorrow:

-
-     _____

Quote of the Day:

-     _____

Day 283:

Date: _____

Mood: _____

Gratitude:

-
-
- _____

Today's Highlights:

-
- _____

Challenges or Struggles:

-
- _____

What I Learned Today:

-
- _____

Dreams:

-
- _____

Goals for Tomorrow:

-
- _____

Quote of the Day:

- _____

Day 284:

Date: _____

Mood: _____

Gratitude:

-
-
-     _____

Today's Highlights:

-
-     _____

Challenges or Struggles:

-
-     _____

What I Learned Today:

-
-     _____

Dreams:

-
-     _____

Goals for Tomorrow:

-
-     _____

Quote of the Day:

-     _____

Day 285:

Date: _____

Mood: _____

Gratitude:

-
-
- _____

Today's Highlights:

-
- _____

Challenges or Struggles:

-
- _____

What I Learned Today:

-
- _____

Dreams:

-
- _____

Goals for Tomorrow:

-
- _____

Quote of the Day:

- _____

Day 286:

Date: _____

Mood: _____

Gratitude:

-
-
- _____

Today's Highlights:

-
- _____

Challenges or Struggles:

-
- _____

What I Learned Today:

-
- _____

Dreams:

-
- _____

Goals for Tomorrow:

-
- _____

Quote of the Day:

- _____

Day 287:

Date: _____

Mood: _____

Gratitude:

-
-
- _____

Today's Highlights:

-
- _____

Challenges or Struggles:

-
- _____

What I Learned Today:

-
- _____

Dreams:

-
- _____

Goals for Tomorrow:

-
- _____

Quote of the Day:

- _____

Day 288:

Date: _____

Mood: _____

Gratitude:

-
-
- _____

Today's Highlights:

-
- _____

Challenges or Struggles:

-
- _____

What I Learned Today:

-
- _____

Dreams:

-
- _____

Goals for Tomorrow:

-
- _____

Quote of the Day:

- _____

Day 289:

Date: _____

Mood: _____

Gratitude:

-
-
- _____

Today's Highlights:

-
- _____

Challenges or Struggles:

-
- _____

What I Learned Today:

-
- _____

Dreams:

-
- _____

Goals for Tomorrow:

-
- _____

Quote of the Day:

- _____

Day 290:

Date: _____

Mood: _____

Gratitude:

-
-
- _____

Today's Highlights:

-
- _____

Challenges or Struggles:

-
- _____

What I Learned Today:

-
- _____

Dreams:

-
- _____

Goals for Tomorrow:

-
- _____

Quote of the Day:

- _____

Day 291:

Date: _____

Mood: _____

Gratitude:

-
-
-    _____

Today's Highlights:

-
-    _____

Challenges or Struggles:

-
-    _____

What I Learned Today:

-
-    _____

Dreams:

-
-    _____

Goals for Tomorrow:

-
-    _____

Quote of the Day:

-    _____

Day 292:

Date: _____

Mood: _____

Gratitude:

-
-
- _____

Today's Highlights:

-
- _____

Challenges or Struggles:

-
- _____

What I Learned Today:

-
- _____

Dreams:

-
- _____

Goals for Tomorrow:

-
- _____

Quote of the Day:

- _____

Day 293:

Date: _____

Mood: _____

Gratitude:

-
-
- _____

Today's Highlights:

-
- _____

Challenges or Struggles:

-
- _____

What I Learned Today:

-
- _____

Dreams:

-
- _____

Goals for Tomorrow:

-
- _____

Quote of the Day:

- _____

Day 294:

Date: _____

Mood: _____

Gratitude:

-
-
-     _____

Today's Highlights:

-
-     _____

Challenges or Struggles:

-
-     _____

What I Learned Today:

-
-     _____

Dreams:

-
-     _____

Goals for Tomorrow:

-
-     _____

Quote of the Day:

-     _____

Day 295:

Date: _____

Mood: _____

Gratitude:

-
-
-    _____

Today's Highlights:

-
-    _____

Challenges or Struggles:

-
-    _____

What I Learned Today:

-
-    _____

Dreams:

-
-    _____

Goals for Tomorrow:

-
-    _____

Quote of the Day:

-    _____

Day 296:

Date: _____

Mood: _____

Gratitude:

-
-
-   _____

Today's Highlights:

-
-   _____

Challenges or Struggles:

-
-   _____

What I Learned Today:

-
-   _____

Dreams:

-
-   _____

Goals for Tomorrow:

-
-   _____

Quote of the Day:

-   _____

Day 297:

Date: _____

Mood: _____

Gratitude:

-
-
- _____

Today's Highlights:

-
- _____

Challenges or Struggles:

-
- _____

What I Learned Today:

-
- _____

Dreams:

-
- _____

Goals for Tomorrow:

-
- _____

Quote of the Day:

- _____

Day 298:

Date: _____

Mood: _____

Gratitude:

-
-
- _____

Today's Highlights:

-
- _____

Challenges or Struggles:

-
- _____

What I Learned Today:

-
- _____

Dreams:

-
- _____

Goals for Tomorrow:

-
- _____

Quote of the Day:

- _____

Day 299:

Date: _____

Mood: _____

Gratitude:

-
-
- _____

Today's Highlights:

-
- _____

Challenges or Struggles:

-
- _____

What I Learned Today:

-
- _____

Dreams:

-
- _____

Goals for Tomorrow:

-
- _____

Quote of the Day:

- _____

Day 300:

Date: _____

Mood: _____

Gratitude:

-
-
- _____

Today's Highlights:

-
- _____

Challenges or Struggles:

-
- _____

What I Learned Today:

-
- _____

Dreams:

-
- _____

Goals for Tomorrow:

-
- _____

Quote of the Day:

- _____

Day 301:

Date: _____

Mood: _____

Gratitude:

-
-
- _____

Today's Highlights:

-
- _____

Challenges or Struggles:

-
- _____

What I Learned Today:

-
- _____

Dreams:

-
- _____

Goals for Tomorrow:

-
- _____

Quote of the Day:

- _____

Day 302:

Date: _____

Mood: _____

Gratitude:

-
-
- _____

Today's Highlights:

-
- _____

Challenges or Struggles:

-
- _____

What I Learned Today:

-
- _____

Dreams:

-
- _____

Goals for Tomorrow:

-
- _____

Quote of the Day:

- _____

Day 303:

Date: _____

Mood: _____

Gratitude:

-
-
- _____

Today's Highlights:

-
- _____

Challenges or Struggles:

-
- _____

What I Learned Today:

-
- _____

Dreams:

-
- _____

Goals for Tomorrow:

-
- _____

Quote of the Day:

- _____

Day 304:

Date: _____

Mood: _____

Gratitude:

-
-
- _____

Today's Highlights:

-
- _____

Challenges or Struggles:

-
- _____

What I Learned Today:

-
- _____

Dreams:

-
- _____

Goals for Tomorrow:

-
- _____

Quote of the Day:

- _____

Day 305:

Date: _____

Mood: _____

Gratitude:

-
-
- _____

Today's Highlights:

-
- _____

Challenges or Struggles:

-
- _____

What I Learned Today:

-
- _____

Dreams:

-
- _____

Goals for Tomorrow:

-
- _____

Quote of the Day:

- _____

Day 306:

Date: _____

Mood: _____

Gratitude:

-
-
- _____

Today's Highlights:

-
- _____

Challenges or Struggles:

-
- _____

What I Learned Today:

-
- _____

Dreams:

-
- _____

Goals for Tomorrow:

-
- _____

Quote of the Day:

- _____
-

Day 307:

Date: _____

Mood: _____

Gratitude:

-
-
- _____

Today's Highlights:

-
- _____

Challenges or Struggles:

-
- _____

What I Learned Today:

-
- _____

Dreams:

-
- _____

Goals for Tomorrow:

-
- _____

Quote of the Day:

- _____

Day 308:

Date: _____

Mood: _____

Gratitude:

-
-
- _____

Today's Highlights:

-
- _____

Challenges or Struggles:

-
- _____

What I Learned Today:

-
- _____

Dreams:

-
- _____

Goals for Tomorrow:

-
- _____

Quote of the Day:

- _____

Day 309:

Date: _____

Mood: _____

Gratitude:

-
-
-    _____

Today's Highlights:

-
-    _____

Challenges or Struggles:

-
-    _____

What I Learned Today:

-
-    _____

Dreams:

-
-    _____

Goals for Tomorrow:

-
-    _____

Quote of the Day:

-    _____

Day 310:

Date: _____

Mood: _____

Gratitude:

-
-
- _____

Today's Highlights:

-
- _____

Challenges or Struggles:

-
- _____

What I Learned Today:

-
- _____

Dreams:

-
- _____

Goals for Tomorrow:

-
- _____

Quote of the Day:

- _____

Day 311:

Date: _____

Mood: _____

Gratitude:

-
-
- _____

Today's Highlights:

-
- _____

Challenges or Struggles:

-
- _____

What I Learned Today:

-
- _____

Dreams:

-
- _____

Goals for Tomorrow:

-
- _____

Quote of the Day:

- _____

Day 312:

Date: _____

Mood: _____

Gratitude:

-
-
- _____

Today's Highlights:

-
- _____

Challenges or Struggles:

-
- _____

What I Learned Today:

-
- _____

Dreams:

-
- _____

Goals for Tomorrow:

-
- _____

Quote of the Day:

- _____

Day 313:

Date: _____

Mood: _____

Gratitude:

-
-
- _____

Today's Highlights:

-
- _____

Challenges or Struggles:

-
- _____

What I Learned Today:

-
- _____

Dreams:

-
- _____

Goals for Tomorrow:

-
- _____

Quote of the Day:

- _____

Day 314:

Date: _____

Mood: _____

Gratitude:

-
-
- _____

Today's Highlights:

-
- _____

Challenges or Struggles:

-
- _____

What I Learned Today:

-
- _____

Dreams:

-
- _____

Goals for Tomorrow:

-
- _____

Quote of the Day:

- _____

Day 315:

Date: _____

Mood: _____

Gratitude:

-
-
- _____

Today's Highlights:

-
- _____

Challenges or Struggles:

-
- _____

What I Learned Today:

-
- _____

Dreams:

-
- _____

Goals for Tomorrow:

-
- _____

Quote of the Day:

- _____

Day 316:

Date: _____

Mood: _____

Gratitude:

-
-
- _____

Today's Highlights:

-
- _____

Challenges or Struggles:

-
- _____

What I Learned Today:

-
- _____

Dreams:

-
- _____

Goals for Tomorrow:

-
- _____

Quote of the Day:

- _____

Day 317:

Date: _____

Mood: _____

Gratitude:

-
-
- _____

Today's Highlights:

-
- _____

Challenges or Struggles:

-
- _____

What I Learned Today:

-
- _____

Dreams:

-
- _____

Goals for Tomorrow:

-
- _____

Quote of the Day:

- _____

Day 318:

Date: _____

Mood: _____

Gratitude:

-
-
-     _____

Today's Highlights:

-
-     _____

Challenges or Struggles:

-
-     _____

What I Learned Today:

-
-     _____

Dreams:

-
-     _____

Goals for Tomorrow:

-
-     _____

Quote of the Day:

-     _____

Day 319:

Date: _____

Mood: _____

Gratitude:

-
-
- _____

Today's Highlights:

-
- _____

Challenges or Struggles:

-
- _____

What I Learned Today:

-
- _____

Dreams:

-
- _____

Goals for Tomorrow:

-
- _____

Quote of the Day:

- _____

Day 320:

Date: _____

Mood: _____

Gratitude:

-
-
- _____

Today's Highlights:

-
- _____

Challenges or Struggles:

-
- _____

What I Learned Today:

-
- _____

Dreams:

-
- _____

Goals for Tomorrow:

-
- _____

Quote of the Day:

- _____

Day 321:

Date: _____

Mood: _____

Gratitude:

-
-
-     _____

Today's Highlights:

-
-     _____

Challenges or Struggles:

-
-     _____

What I Learned Today:

-
-     _____

Dreams:

-
-     _____

Goals for Tomorrow:

-
-     _____

Quote of the Day:

-     _____

Day 322:

Date: _____

Mood: _____

Gratitude:

-
-
- _____

Today's Highlights:

-
- _____

Challenges or Struggles:

-
- _____

What I Learned Today:

-
- _____

Dreams:

-
- _____

Goals for Tomorrow:

-
- _____

Quote of the Day:

- _____

Day 323:

Date: _____

Mood: _____

Gratitude:

-
-
-    _____

Today's Highlights:

-
-    _____

Challenges or Struggles:

-
-    _____

What I Learned Today:

-
-    _____

Dreams:

-
-    _____

Goals for Tomorrow:

-
-    _____

Quote of the Day:

-    _____

Day 324:

Date: _____

Mood: _____

Gratitude:

-
-
-    _____

Today's Highlights:

-
-    _____

Challenges or Struggles:

-
-    _____

What I Learned Today:

-
-    _____

Dreams:

-
-    _____

Goals for Tomorrow:

-
-    _____

Quote of the Day:

-    _____

Day 325:

Date: _____

Mood: _____

Gratitude:

-
-
- _____

Today's Highlights:

-
- _____

Challenges or Struggles:

-
- _____

What I Learned Today:

-
- _____

Dreams:

-
- _____

Goals for Tomorrow:

-
- _____

Quote of the Day:

- _____

Day 326:

Date: _____

Mood: _____

Gratitude:

-
-
-      _____

Today's Highlights:

-
-      _____

Challenges or Struggles:

-
-      _____

What I Learned Today:

-
-      _____

Dreams:

-
-      _____

Goals for Tomorrow:

-
-      _____

Quote of the Day:

-      _____

Day 327:

Date: _____

Mood: _____

Gratitude:

-
-
- _____

Today's Highlights:

-
- _____

Challenges or Struggles:

-
- _____

What I Learned Today:

-
- _____

Dreams:

-
- _____

Goals for Tomorrow:

-
- _____

Quote of the Day:

- _____

Day 328:

Date: _____

Mood: _____

Gratitude:

-
-
- _____

Today's Highlights:

-
- _____

Challenges or Struggles:

-
- _____

What I Learned Today:

-
- _____

Dreams:

-
- _____

Goals for Tomorrow:

-
- _____

Quote of the Day:

- _____

Day 329:

Date: _____

Mood: _____

Gratitude:

-
-
- _____

Today's Highlights:

-
- _____

Challenges or Struggles:

-
- _____

What I Learned Today:

-
- _____

Dreams:

-
- _____

Goals for Tomorrow:

-
- _____

Quote of the Day:

- _____

Day 330:

Date: _____

Mood: _____

Gratitude:

-
-
- _____

Today's Highlights:

-
- _____

Challenges or Struggles:

-
- _____

What I Learned Today:

-
- _____

Dreams:

-
- _____

Goals for Tomorrow:

-
- _____

Quote of the Day:

- _____

Day 331:

Date: _____

Mood: _____

Gratitude:

-
-
- _____

Today's Highlights:

-
- _____

Challenges or Struggles:

-
- _____

What I Learned Today:

-
- _____

Dreams:

-
- _____

Goals for Tomorrow:

-
- _____

Quote of the Day:

- _____

Day 332:

Date: _____

Mood: _____

Gratitude:

-
-
- _____

Today's Highlights:

-
- _____

Challenges or Struggles:

-
- _____

What I Learned Today:

-
- _____

Dreams:

-
- _____

Goals for Tomorrow:

-
- _____

Quote of the Day:

- _____

Day 333:

Date: _____

Mood: _____

Gratitude:

-
-
- _____

Today's Highlights:

-
- _____

Challenges or Struggles:

-
- _____

What I Learned Today:

-
- _____

Dreams:

-
- _____

Goals for Tomorrow:

-
- _____

Quote of the Day:

- _____

Day 334:

Date: _____

Mood: _____

Gratitude:

-
-
- _____

Today's Highlights:

-
- _____

Challenges or Struggles:

-
- _____

What I Learned Today:

-
- _____

Dreams:

-
- _____

Goals for Tomorrow:

-
- _____

Quote of the Day:

- _____

Day 335:

Date: _____

Mood: _____

Gratitude:

-
-
- _____

Today's Highlights:

-
- _____

Challenges or Struggles:

-
- _____

What I Learned Today:

-
- _____

Dreams:

-
- _____

Goals for Tomorrow:

-
- _____

Quote of the Day:

- _____

Day 336:

Date: _____

Mood: _____

Gratitude:

-
-
- _____

Today's Highlights:

-
- _____

Challenges or Struggles:

-
- _____

What I Learned Today:

-
- _____

Dreams:

-
- _____

Goals for Tomorrow:

-
- _____

Quote of the Day:

- _____

Day 337:

Date: _____

Mood: _____

Gratitude:

-
-
- _____

Today's Highlights:

-
- _____

Challenges or Struggles:

-
- _____

What I Learned Today:

-
- _____

Dreams:

-
- _____

Goals for Tomorrow:

-
- _____

Quote of the Day:

- _____

Day 338:

Date: _____

Mood: _____

Gratitude:

-
-
- _____

Today's Highlights:

-
- _____

Challenges or Struggles:

-
- _____

What I Learned Today:

-
- _____

Dreams:

-
- _____

Goals for Tomorrow:

-
- _____

Quote of the Day:

- _____

Day 339:

Date: _____

Mood: _____

Gratitude:

-
-
- _____

Today's Highlights:

-
- _____

Challenges or Struggles:

-
- _____

What I Learned Today:

-
- _____

Dreams:

-
- _____

Goals for Tomorrow:

-
- _____

Quote of the Day:

- _____

Day 340:

Date: _____

Mood: _____

Gratitude:

-
-
- _____

Today's Highlights:

-
- _____

Challenges or Struggles:

-
- _____

What I Learned Today:

-
- _____

Dreams:

-
- _____

Goals for Tomorrow:

-
- _____

Quote of the Day:

- _____

Day 341:

Date: _____

Mood: _____

Gratitude:

-
-
- _____

Today's Highlights:

-
- _____

Challenges or Struggles:

-
- _____

What I Learned Today:

-
- _____

Dreams:

-
- _____

Goals for Tomorrow:

-
- _____

Quote of the Day:

- _____

Day 342:

Date: _____

Mood: _____

Gratitude:

-
-
-       _____

Today's Highlights:

-
-       _____

Challenges or Struggles:

-
-       _____

What I Learned Today:

-
-       _____

Dreams:

-
-       _____

Goals for Tomorrow:

-
-       _____

Quote of the Day:

-       _____

Day 343:

Date: _____

Mood: _____

Gratitude:

-
-
- _____

Today's Highlights:

-
- _____

Challenges or Struggles:

-
- _____

What I Learned Today:

-
- _____

Dreams:

-
- _____

Goals for Tomorrow:

-
- _____

Quote of the Day:

- _____

Day 344:

Date: _____

Mood: _____

Gratitude:

-
-
- _____

Today's Highlights:

-
- _____

Challenges or Struggles:

-
- _____

What I Learned Today:

-
- _____

Dreams:

-
- _____

Goals for Tomorrow:

-
- _____

Quote of the Day:

- _____

Day 345:

Date: _____

Mood: _____

Gratitude:

-
-
- _____

Today's Highlights:

-
- _____

Challenges or Struggles:

-
- _____

What I Learned Today:

-
- _____

Dreams:

-
- _____

Goals for Tomorrow:

-
- _____

Quote of the Day:

- _____

Day 346:

Date: _____

Mood: _____

Gratitude:

-
-
- _____

Today's Highlights:

-
- _____

Challenges or Struggles:

-
- _____

What I Learned Today:

-
- _____

Dreams:

-
- _____

Goals for Tomorrow:

-
- _____

Quote of the Day:

- _____

Day 347:

Date: _____

Mood: _____

Gratitude:

-
-
- _____

Today's Highlights:

-
- _____

Challenges or Struggles:

-
- _____

What I Learned Today:

-
- _____

Dreams:

-
- _____

Goals for Tomorrow:

-
- _____

Quote of the Day:

- _____

Day 348:

Date: _____

Mood: _____

Gratitude:

-
-
- _____

Today's Highlights:

-
- _____

Challenges or Struggles:

-
- _____

What I Learned Today:

-
- _____

Dreams:

-
- _____

Goals for Tomorrow:

-
- _____

Quote of the Day:

- _____

Day 349:

Date: _____

Mood: _____

Gratitude:

-
-
- _____

Today's Highlights:

-
- _____

Challenges or Struggles:

-
- _____

What I Learned Today:

-
- _____

Dreams:

-
- _____

Goals for Tomorrow:

-
- _____

Quote of the Day:

- _____

Day 350:

Date: _____

Mood: _____

Gratitude:

-
-
- _____

Today's Highlights:

-
- _____

Challenges or Struggles:

-
- _____

What I Learned Today:

-
- _____

Dreams:

-
- _____

Goals for Tomorrow:

-
- _____

Quote of the Day:

- _____

Day 351:

Date: _____

Mood: _____

Gratitude:

-
-
-   _____

Today's Highlights:

-
-   _____

Challenges or Struggles:

-
-   _____

What I Learned Today:

-
-   _____

Dreams:

-
-   _____

Goals for Tomorrow:

-
-   _____

Quote of the Day:

-   _____

Day 352:

Date: _____

Mood: _____

Gratitude:

-
-
- _____

Today's Highlights:

-
- _____

Challenges or Struggles:

-
- _____

What I Learned Today:

-
- _____

Dreams:

-
- _____

Goals for Tomorrow:

-
- _____

Quote of the Day:

- _____

Day 353:

Date: _____

Mood: _____

Gratitude:

-
-
- _____

Today's Highlights:

-
- _____

Challenges or Struggles:

-
- _____

What I Learned Today:

-
- _____

Dreams:

-
- _____

Goals for Tomorrow:

-
- _____

Quote of the Day:

- _____

Day 354:

Date: _____

Mood: _____

Gratitude:

-
-
- _____

Today's Highlights:

-
- _____

Challenges or Struggles:

-
- _____

What I Learned Today:

-
- _____

Dreams:

-
- _____

Goals for Tomorrow:

-
- _____

Quote of the Day:

- _____

Day 355:

Date: _____
Mood: _____

Gratitude:

-
-
- _____

Today's Highlights:

-
- _____

Challenges or Struggles:

-
- _____

What I Learned Today:

-
- _____

Dreams:

-
- _____

Goals for Tomorrow:

-
- _____

Quote of the Day:

- _____

Day 356:

Date: _____

Mood: _____

Gratitude:

-
-
-     _____

Today's Highlights:

-
-     _____

Challenges or Struggles:

-
-     _____

What I Learned Today:

-
-     _____

Dreams:

-
-     _____

Goals for Tomorrow:

-
-     _____

Quote of the Day:

-     _____

Day 357:

Date: _____

Mood: _____

Gratitude:

-
-
- _____

Today's Highlights:

-
- _____

Challenges or Struggles:

-
- _____

What I Learned Today:

-
- _____

Dreams:

-
- _____

Goals for Tomorrow:

-
- _____

Quote of the Day:

- _____

Day 358:

Date: _____

Mood: _____

Gratitude:

-
-
- _____

Today's Highlights:

-
- _____

Challenges or Struggles:

-
- _____

What I Learned Today:

-
- _____

Dreams:

-
- _____

Goals for Tomorrow:

-
- _____

Quote of the Day:

- _____

Day 359:

Date: _____

Mood: _____

Gratitude:

-
-
- _____

Today's Highlights:

-
- _____

Challenges or Struggles:

-
- _____

What I Learned Today:

-
- _____

Dreams:

-
- _____

Goals for Tomorrow:

-
- _____

Quote of the Day:

- _____

Day 360:

Date: _____

Mood: _____

Gratitude:

-
-
- _____

Today's Highlights:

-
- _____

Challenges or Struggles:

-
- _____

What I Learned Today:

-
- _____

Dreams:

-
- _____

Goals for Tomorrow:

-
- _____

Quote of the Day:

- _____

Day 361:

Date: _____

Mood: _____

Gratitude:

-
-
- _____

Today's Highlights:

-
- _____

Challenges or Struggles:

-
- _____

What I Learned Today:

-
- _____

Dreams:

-
- _____

Goals for Tomorrow:

-
- _____

Quote of the Day:

- _____

Day 362:

Date: _____

Mood: _____

Gratitude:

-
-
- _____

Today's Highlights:

-
- _____

Challenges or Struggles:

-
- _____

What I Learned Today:

-
- _____

Dreams:

-
- _____

Goals for Tomorrow:

-
- _____

Quote of the Day:

- _____

Day 363:

Date: _____

Mood: _____

Gratitude:

-
-
- _____

Today's Highlights:

-
- _____

Challenges or Struggles:

-
- _____

What I Learned Today:

-
- _____

Dreams:

-
- _____

Goals for Tomorrow:

-
- _____

Quote of the Day:

- _____

Day 364:

Date: _____

Mood: _____

Gratitude:

-
-
- _____

Today's Highlights:

-
- _____

Challenges or Struggles:

-
- _____

What I Learned Today:

-
- _____

Dreams:

-
- _____

Goals for Tomorrow:

-
- _____

Quote of the Day:

- _____

Day 365:

Date: _____

Mood: _____

Gratitude:

-
-
- _____

Today's Highlights:

-
- _____

Challenges or Struggles:

-
- _____

What I Learned Today:

-
- _____

Dreams:

-
- _____

Goals for Tomorrow:

-
- _____

Quote of the Day:

- _____

Notes:

Notes:

Notes:

Notes:

Notes:

Notes:

Notes:

Notes:

Notes:

Notes:

Notes:

Notes:

Notes:

Notes:

Notes:

Notes:

Notes:

Notes:

Notes:

Notes:

Notes:

_____
_____
_____
_____
_____
_____
_____
_____
_____
_____
_____
_____
_____
_____
_____
_____
_____
_____
_____
_____
_____
_____
_____
_____
_____
_____
_____
_____

Notes:

Notes:

Notes:

Notes:

Notes:

Notes:

Notes:

Notes:

Notes:

Notes:

Notes:

Notes:

Notes:

Notes:

Notes:

Notes:

Notes:

Notes:

Notes:

Notes:

Notes:

Notes:

Notes:

Notes:

Notes:

Notes:

Notes:

Notes:

Notes:

Notes:

Notes:

Notes:

Notes:

Notes:

Notes:

Notes:

Notes:

Notes:

Notes:

Notes:

Notes:

Notes:

Notes:

Notes:

Notes:

Notes:

Notes:

Notes:

Notes:

_____

_____

_____

_____

_____

_____

_____

_____

_____

_____

_____

_____

_____

_____

_____

_____

_____

_____

_____

_____

_____

_____

_____

_____

_____

_____

_____

Notes:

Notes:

Notes:

Notes:

Notes:

Notes:

Notes:

Notes:

_____

_____

_____

_____

_____

_____

_____

_____

_____

_____

_____

_____

_____

_____

_____

_____

_____

_____

_____

_____

_____

_____

_____

_____

_____

_____

_____

Notes:

Notes:

Notes:

Notes:

Notes:

Notes:

Notes:

Notes:

Notes:

Notes:

Notes:

Notes: